To everyone that helped me walk again.

First Edition

ISBN-13: 978-1503202894

ISBN-10: 1503202895

PRINTED IN THE UNITED STATES OF AMERICA

Medical Disclaimer

The information in this book is not intended or implied to be a substitute for professional medical advice, diagnosis or treatment. All content, including text, graphics, images and information, contained on or available through this book is for general information purposes only. The author makes no representation and assumes no responsibility for the accuracy of information contained on or available through this book, and such information is subject to change without notice. You are encouraged to confirm any information obtained from or through this book with other sources, and review all information regarding any medical condition or treatment with your physician.

NEVER DISREGARD PROFESSIONAL MEDICAL ADVICE OR DELAY SEEKING MEDICAL TREATMENT BECAUSE OF SOMETHING YOU HAVE READ ON OR ACCESSED THROUGH THIS BOOK.

The author does not recommend, endorse or make any representation about the efficacy, appropriateness or suitability of any specific tests, products, procedures, treatments, services, opinions, health care providers or other information that may be contained on or available through this book.

THE AUTHORS IS NEITHER RESPONSIBLE NOR LIABLE FOR ANY ADVICE, COURSE OF TREATMENT, DIAGNOSIS OR ANY OTHER INFORMATION, SERVICES OR PRODUCTS THAT YOU OBTAIN THROUGH THIS BOOK."

Affiliation and Endorsement Disclaimer

Any product names, logos, brands, and other trademarks or images featured or referred to within this book are the property of their respective trademark holders. These trademark holders are not affiliated with the author, this book, or our website. They do not sponsor or endorse the chronic injury survival guide or any of our online products. The chronic injury survival guide declares no affiliation, sponsorship, nor any partnerships with any registered trademarks.

Table of Contents

SECOND STEP OF MSTR:

THIRD STEP OF MSTR: KINETIC CHAIN STRETCHES

SPINAL KINETIC STRETCHES   167

KINETIC CHAIN STRETCHES FOR THE REST OF THE BODY   174

How to Fix the Unfixable

Are you in pain? Did the pain start from a simple injury then get worse as time went on? Did you see your doctor and all he/she could say was "Try icing it, maybe use some NSAIDs and rest the area" and send you on your way? For many of us, these directions lead to a dead end of pain and painkillers.

I know this frustration personally. I have had to deal with it for years. There was a point when I could not walk for 5 months straight; at another time, I had my arm in a sling for 2 months, unable to use it. After following the basic "treatment advice" that doctors gave me and not seeing good results, I started to read about alternative therapies. I found things that worked, and that is what got me out of the wheel chair.

This book is made to fix your chronic injuries, but it is going to take some work. You are your own best therapist. You must understand that when you see a doctor, you cannot expect them to miraculously fix your pain on the spot. If they tried to fix your pain with drugs, then they probably ignored the causes of the pain.

This book is made to give you insight into what is perpetuating your pain, and what you can do to fix it. I will take the time to show you what is going on, and why your body is unable to heal from the damage.

This book is made to show you step by step instructions on what to do for a variety of chronic injuries that are common today. When injuries become chronic, they do not just "heal". They are usually degenerative and in a downward spiral, slowly getting worse and/or spreading to other areas of the body. Most doctors will not understand how much pain you have and just simply write you a prescription for pain medication. This does not solve anything. Let's fix the pain and move on with our lives!

How Chronic Pain Injuries Start and How They are Perpetuated

In order to understand how chronic injuries happen, let's first go over what happens when you have a normal injury.

The Events of a Normal Injury

When you have a normal injury anywhere in your body, your body responds with inflammation. This causes a cascade of events that are triggered by the chemicals that produce inflammation:

1. The area becomes hot and inflamed (red and swollen, this is to rush nutrients into the area).

2. Tenderness at the site of the injury occurs (pain when touched).

3. The muscles around the injury tighten up (to splint the area and to force rest).

4. The Fascia (connective tissue around the muscle fibers) also tightens up to splint the injury.

5. Movement of the joints around the injury becomes restricted due to the tight muscles and fascia.

When this happens, the body is telling the injured person to rest. Usually, guided by pain, we are forced to rest the area, and in a couple of days to a few weeks, the injury heals, the muscles relax and loosen, the swelling goes away, the tenderness subsides, and we regain all of our flexibility. It may hurt a bit for a while, but it is usually "live-able" pain. We notice it, but it is manageable. In a couple months, that pain slowly disappears, and we are all healed up.

The Events of an Unhealthy and Chronic Injury

The events mentioned above all happen. But the big difference that makes a normal injury turn into a chronic one is that most people have to keep on working/going to school/taking care of the kids. Most people love to "push through the pain". If you combine this mentality with an unhealthy diet, you are putting yourself at risk for chronic injuries.

When the body tells you to rest, but you keep on moving through the pain and using pain killers when the pain becomes unbearable, you are damaging your body severely. When you use pain killers, you do not feel the pain that you need to feel. Pain is very important; its purpose is to tell you what not to do. Ignoring the pain will make the pain worse later on.

The above applies to most severe onset injuries as well. Not resting and continuing to push through the pain is horrible for these kinds of injuries. If 6-8 weeks pass by and you're still in pain, you now have chronic inflammation. This is when healing stops, and the body "gives up" on healing the injury. It starts to break the area down and it slowly becomes weaker and weaker. Eventually, the injured structures start to break or ruptures; then you are unable to use that area of the body, forcing you to rest.

Another way to get chronic pain injuries is by having bad posture while sitting, standing, and moving. A lot of people live sedentary lives where they are stuck in one position all day long. When this happens, the body says "ok, you want to sit down all day? I am going to shorten a couple muscles here and there and make this whole 'sitting' thing easier for you". When your body responds in this way, it puts your body out of its natural alignment. When your posture is out of place, and no longer in a stable position to withstand the forces acted upon it, it breaks down.

All of our joints need to rotate and bend within their natural range of motion to make them stable and strong. When your muscles and other bodily structures tighten up to make, for example, "sitting", easier, it causes problems. Your body was not designed to sit all day long. You were not made to type on a keyboard, hunched over a computer screen for 8 hours a day. You were not made to stand at a checkout stand and do the same repetitive tasks over and over for hours on end. Your body is made to be outside, moving all day long. We are made to walk without restricting shoes. When you take an animal such as ourselves, and stick them in a chair, in uncomfortable shoes, or in a car (which is far from natural), you are causing problems.

When the body is in compromising positions like sitting, the joints are not in their ideal position to be strong. This means over time, when the joint adapts to the new position, the joint will become unstable. When a joint is not in a strong and stable position, problems arise. An unstable joint is just asking for injury because it is extremely weak.

Muscles stabilize joints. The muscles also act as shock absorbers. If the muscles that control a joint are firing in a dysfunctional way (usually from having trigger points), the joints associated with said muscles will become unstable as well (and unable to absorb the shock from the forces acted upon them).

How do the muscles become functionally unable to stabilize a joint? This occurs from having a severe injury; from damage done to a joint from being in compromising positions over the course of months (or sometimes years); or from doing the same task over and over for hours on end. Once the muscles are dysfunctional and causing damage to the joints, the joints respond with a chemical response telling the muscles to stay dysfunctional. This is the downward spiral that this book aims to fix.

When a muscle has been dysfunctional for 6-8 weeks, the connective tissue cells around the muscle start to lay down scar tissue. This scar tissue is called "cross-link adhesions". These are the body's natural adaptations to the new stressors imposed on the dysfunctional movement patterns associated with having dysfunctional joint dynamics and dysfunctional muscle activity. This is the body's attempt at "splinting" the area.

Connective tissue surrounds every muscle in the body. It literally encapsulates each muscle and is continuous with the tendon that the muscle is attached to, and continuous with the bone the tendon is attached to. Everything in the body is connected with connective tissue. This connective tissue is called fascia. The cross-link adhesions mentioned earlier are created in the fascia. These cross-link adhesions can form anywhere, but the ones we will be talking a lot about are the ones that form around a muscles belly, which causes lots of long-term problems.

Within this connective tissue (fascia) lives what's called "Muscle Spindles" and "Golgi Tendon Organs". What these little sensory organs do is tell your brain centers how much stress is being imposed on the tendons and muscles. They tell your brain how far you have raised your arm, or how long your stride is. These little sensory organs are responsible for telling your body where your body is in 3 dimensional space.

If too many cross-link adhesions form in the connective tissue, than the sensory organs start giving your brain the wrong signals (this means your body is confused as to where you are in 3 dimensional space). This causes the muscles to fire in ways they're not supposed to. This leads to MORE joint stabilization dysfunction, which means more damage and more pain!

Also, you must remember that another implication to having these cross-link adhesions in the connective tissue surrounding the muscles is that the muscle starts to get a mild form of "compartment syndrome". Because of the encapsulating nature of the connective tissue, and the fact that muscles need to expand in order to contract, the connective tissue must be fluid and able to move and slide freely past other nearby connective tissue structures. When the cross-link adhesions cause excessive compartment pressure (from putting scar tissue down all over the muscle), or when the muscle is tacked down to nearby structures and unable to slide past other structures, the muscle is unable to contract fully (Or is greatly hindered).

We must always remember that muscles are like pumps and rely on their moving/contracting ability to get nutrients in and out. When the muscle is physically hindered from enlarging due to these cross-link adhesions, the muscle is unable to efficiently push nutrients in and waste out. This causes stagnation in the muscle and promotes the dysfunctional muscle dynamics mentioned earlier (more pain and more trigger points).

Another implication to dysfunctional muscle dynamics is the fact that when a muscle becomes dysfunctional (and harbors trigger points), the muscle is usually in a "chronic spasm". This means that it is always contracted in some areas. You usually feel these as "knots" in the muscle. They can be pea sized lumps or long, taut bands of muscle tissue. When these knots are in the muscle, they cause lots of issues.

When a trigger point (or knot) is causing a chronic spasm of the muscle, the muscle is unable to do its job of "pumping" nutrients and wastes in and out of the muscle. This leads to stagnation in the muscle, which leads to the hardening of fluids in and around the muscle cell. They go from being liquid and healthy, to gel-like and dysfunctional.

When a trigger point has been around for a while, and stagnation has set in, nerve irritant chemicals (bradykinin, serotonin etc.) get secreted by cells nearby, and cause more pain and perpetuate the problem even further.

After a while, the nerves that pass through and around the muscles and connective tissue become entrapped and entangled in the scar tissue that has been laid down around the injury. This is when you get all sorts of nerve issues including numbness, burning, and more pain.

If you can stop this cycle and fix the causes, the pain will disappear!

So to summarize this whole process:

1. Severe injury/Bad posture/Sedentary lifestyle causes damage or mis-alignment to an area of the body.

2. The body uses trigger points to splint the area and joints associated with the area so that you do not move the area. Your body is trying to say "if you move this joint, I am going to make it hurt!"

3. Trigger points cause localized stagnation/joint instability (this is ok short term, but not long-term).

4. A person in pain usually has to work/take care of kids etc, so they usually take pain pills at this point and/or push through the pain. Lots of mental frustration and confusion sets in because pain seems permanent and rules the person's thoughts. Lots of "is this going to ever get better?" and "why me?" thoughts arise.

5. Because they push through the pain while trigger points are in the muscles, more damage occurs (an unstable joint is a weak joint, doing daily activities with an unstable joint can cause serious damage). After 6-8 weeks, the body gives up on healing, and the area becomes degenerative. This is when the horrible downward spiral occurs.

6. At this point, we start to see scar tissue form in structures around the injury, in the form of cross-link adhesions around the muscles associated with the damaged or dysfunctional joints. These adhesions cause a lost range of motion, further stagnation and more pain.

7. More time passes by and adhesions form in the tubes that carry the nerves (nerves travel in tunnels made from fascia). This causes numbness/burning pain/weakness etc.

8. Muscles are still dysfunctional and chronically contracted from the trigger points; this hinders nutrient/waste exchange and further perpetuates the problem.

9. Eventually, this downward spiral continues until you cannot move the area.

How Do We Stop The Chronic Inflammatory Cycle?

With MSTR! I have created a way to fix the causes and perpetuating factors that happen in a chronic inflammatory injury.

Most of what my therapy does is use common and practical therapies that are practiced and proven for their efficacy, then combined in a way to fix chronic injuries faster than ever before. There are three crucial components to MSTR:

1. Get rid of the trigger points in the muscular system. This will get rid of most of the pain and bring back function to the previously damaged muscles.

2. Break up adhesions in the fascia system. Earlier I talked about cross-link adhesions, and these are what we need to "release". These can only be effectively released when the trigger points are long gone.

3. Use Kinetic Chain Stretches to elongate the fascia in a way that the trigger points and fascia adhesions do not come back. These stretches are made to not stress the muscles; they are made to stretch the fascia (connective tissue) that encapsulates the muscles.

Why are we doing it in this order? Simply because they work much better in this sequence than otherwise. Another thing we need to address is what in your daily life actually caused the pain? What movement patterns have you adopted in your daily life that is perpetuating your pain? We will get into this more later, after the pain is gone and we are trying to keep the pain away for the long-term.

First off, a trigger point is muscular dysfunction, a chronic contraction of a select set of muscle fibers. They have quite a few characteristics that make them important to address first and foremost before using other therapy methods. Some of the most crucial reasons are:

• They cause pain in weird ways. You can have a trigger point harbored in a muscle near the neck causing pain in the hand. Most of the pain we feel in chronic pain injuries stems from these "referred pain patterns". It simply means that one area of trigger point dysfunction is causing pain elsewhere in the body. (This does not hold true if you have a chronic injury and certain pain syndromes such as RSD/fibromyalgia or any other pain syndromes known today.)

• The trigger point stops the muscles from doing their job of "pumping". This causes the cells to go from a liquid and fluid cell environment to a sticky and hardened environment. When the cells are hardened and sticky, it makes it EXTREMELY hard to break up the adhesions in and around the fascia system. Once you get rid of a trigger point, breaking up the fascial adhesions associated with the trigger point is much easier.

- We need joint stability immediately. If there are any trigger points causing joint stability dysfunction, the joints are in danger. We need to release the trigger points first so that the muscles nearby fire properly and keep the joint strong and stable.

- If the trigger points are so bad that they cause lost range of motion for a joint, then we are in big trouble. Once a joint cannot move how it is made to move, other areas of the body need to adjust for this loss. When nearby joints and muscles are all compensating for the dysfunctional joints immobility, they become damaged as well. We need all the joints to move and rotate together to work efficiently and properly. If this does not happen, dysfunction spreads to other areas of the body and puts the body in a downward spiral, causing more and more pain and dysfunction.

- Nerve irritants are made and perpetuated by trigger point activity. Pain is good and important, but trigger points can cause "too much pain" from the chemical nerve irritants that they promote. This much pain can also cause a lot of stress, which is horrible for our well-being and hormone balance. Too much stress can cause a wide array of issues.

Trigger points are easily taken care of by finding out which muscles are dysfunctional (by following pain referral patterns or by simply feeling the muscles). Then you search for the tender area in the muscle. This is the trigger point, and there are special ways to massage these in order to get them to release.

After we get rid of the muscular systems' trigger point dysfunction, the muscle cells and surrounding cellular environment will not be nearly as "hardened" or "sticky". This means that the next step in MSTR can be carried out. The reason we need to wait until the cells and cell environments are more "fluid" and "softened" is because if you want to break up the cross-link adhesions in the fascia, you need to put a certain amount of mechanical pressure, in a special way, into the fascia system. Ideally, we would like to go in and break up these adhesions by pulling on both sides of each piece of dysfunctional fascia and rip the adhesions apart. This is impossible due to how the body responds to active and forced stretching. The muscle would respond with more dysfunction if you just simply tried to "stretch" out these adhesions. This would make things worse and the fascia system would start laying down more scar tissue (which we do not want!).

The best way to break up these cross-link adhesions in the muscle is by scraping the dysfunctional muscle with certain tools. These tools are much more aggressive than your hands could ever be, and they go in deep due to having a smaller surface area than your hands. They cause the cross-link adhesions to stretch and break.

The fascia system also has a little known contractile effect. This only happens when it has been in a dysfunctional state for a long time. When you break up the cross-link adhesions (which are the structural hindrance to free movement), you also release the contraction of the fascia.

The reason we can release the fascia systems' contractile state is because of mechanoreceptors: sensory organs that live in the fascia system and tell the body where it is in 3 dimensional space. Earlier, we talked about these sensory organs, which are called "muscle spindles" and "golgi tendon organs". The mechanoreceptors lie in the most superficial layers of the fascia system (this means they are close to the skin). When you stimulate these sensory organs with mechanical pressure, such as scraping the area with a cross-link adhesion tool, the fascias' contraction will release. Later in the book we will refer to these tools as "scraping tools".

Remember that the fascia system holds the muscles and organ systems in place. It is also what tendons and ligaments are made from, and is continuous with the 3 dimensional matrix of collagen framework in every single bone in your body. The fascia system connects literally everything in the body! If one small area is contracted, it will be felt across the whole body because of the all-encompassing nature of fascia.

An example of this contractile state of fascia that is commonly used in literature is the sacrotuberous ligament, a huge ligament that connects your sit bones to your sacrum. If you were to dissect the layers of this strong and thick ligament, you will find that all the mechanoreceptors are on the sides closer to the skin (more superficial). Once these are stimulated by scraping the superficial layers, the ligament as a whole "releases". This is a subtle contraction, and the release is not as severe or extreme as a muscular contraction release. It can still perpetuate the pain and needs to be addressed.

After we have addressed the trigger points and fascia adhesions (and contractions), and have gotten rid of most of the pain, we then use kinetic chain stretches to prevent the pain from coming back (and address the biomechanical and structural problems that have developed from having the injury). Kinetic chain stretches are not the same as normal stretches.

When you do regular stretches, by isolating one muscle at a time – especially in a muscle with trigger points – damage can occur (which is why I feel that physical therapists should not prescribe these kinds of stretches). You should not stretch until the trigger points are dealt with before hand. Muscles usually do not need to be "stretched" in order to make them more functional or have less pain. What you do want to stretch is the fascia between the muscles.

In your body, fascia is literally everywhere. But the interesting thing to note about fascia is that there are certain functional "chains" of it throughout the body. The first example I will bring to mind is the SBL (superficial back line). This chain of fascia (and associated muscles in this chain) starts from the toes, goes up the back of your legs, up your back, and ends on the forehead.

This train of fascia starts at the foot flexors and plantar fascia, then wrap around the heel of the foot and become continuous with the calf muscle. The calf muscle makes its way up to the next joint, the knee joint. This is because one of the calf muscles goes from the heel all the way up to the femur bone, thus making it a multi joint muscle. This chain continues upward with the hamstrings.

A couple of the hamstring muscles are multi joint muscles and lie over the knee joint and the hip joint. We then follow the fascia chain further upward, to the ischial tuberosity (the boney lumps you sit on). The connective tissue goes into this bone and further upward to a huge ligament that connects your ischial tuberosity to your sacrum. We continue further upward to the extensors of the back and neck, then to the back of the head. The fascia continues over the head and to the forehead.

In summary, the SBL fascia chain is comprised of:

- Foot muscles that touch the floor (ones that flex toes and support foots arch)

- Calf muscles that cross the knee and ankle joints

- Hamstrings that cross the knee and hip joints

- Sacrotuberous ligament connects hamstring and back muscles

- Back erector muscles

- Back of neck muscles

- Connective tissue continues upward, over the skull and to the forehead

If you were to try to stretch this fascia chain because you have dysfunction anywhere in the chain, you would need to stretch every part of the chain at the same time. This makes it so that the joints associated with the chain stay in their natural range of motion. We do not want to stretch to the point where a joint is out of its strong and stable range of motion. We just need to stretch it enough to undo the bad effects of our chronic injury. We also do not want or need to stretch the muscles (you fix muscle dysfunction with trigger point massage). We use kinetic chain stretches to keep the muscles nice and happy and in their natural range of motion, but we do cause tension in the fascia system so that it can regain its previously functional state.

Fascia is very plastic and taffy like. Once you "reset" your fascia by keeping it held in the position it needs to be in (from kinetic chain stretches), it stays that way. For some people, dysfunctional fascia can be the reason they had the pain in the first place. When a kinetic chain is stuck in one position for an extended amount of time (such as from sitting around all day), the fascia likes to adapt to the new position. Even if the fascia is to blame (and caused the problems), we need to take care of the trigger points first!

There are quite a few chains of fascia in the body. You will fix all the dysfunctional chains in the kinetic chain stretches section later on.

Also, remember that if there is a traumatic or chronic injury in a fascia chain, then the whole chain will be slightly affected. The fascia likes to communicate with itself through chemicals and small electrical currents (in the range of micro-amps), and if there is damage, the whole chain will respond to the damage.

To summarize the basic process of MSTR:

- Get rid of trigger points

- Get rid of fascia adhesions (cross-link adhesions)

- Stop the pain and dysfunction from coming back with kinetic chain stretches

Additional Therapies to Boost Your Results

MSTR is the foundation of my soft tissue mobilization therapy, but there are tons of other therapies that should be used alongside with my therapy. I do not like when therapists become biased to their own methods and ignore other methods that work just as well. Some therapies work better for different injuries. In the section of this book that deals with applying MSTR to individual injuries, I will also show you which additional therapies can help boost your results.

- **Graston®**: My favorite soft tissue mobilization method. If you want to know what it feels like to break up cross-link adhesions and scar tissue, find a therapist in your area that specializes in this technique and go for at least 4 sessions. The doctors I know who practice this therapy are all very smart and know a great deal about soft tissue injuries. I cannot recommend them more.

- **Active Release Technique®**: Releases entrapped nerves, promotes lymphatic flow, and releases adhesions in the soft tissue to speed up healing. Well-studied and will give you great results. Great for chronic and severe injuries. Find a therapist that specializes in your body area (some are better with legs or arms etc) and visit them for at least 4 sessions.

- **ESWT (Extra Corporeal Shockwave Therapy)**: Great for chronic injuries. Causes a localized spot of inflammation which causes the body to work extra hard to fix the damage, and fast. I recommend having ONLY low level or low energy shockwave machines. They give you better results and faster healing times and are much cheaper to use than the more powerful machines (powerful is not better in this situation). Have at least 3 sessions and only use this treatment method for the injuries recommended in the individual injury section.

- **ASTYM®**: Great for chronic injuries which have caused adhesions in the fascia chains. Similar to Graston ® but not quite the same. If you have had pain for more than 6 weeks, it will help you a lot. Go for at least 3 sessions.

- **Cross Friction Massage**: Great for scar tissue. Painful, but very effective. You need a doctor/therapist that is good at this to see results. I had horrible results with a physical therapist doing this at first. Later, I went to a soft tissue specialist, and it hurt 100 times more, but I had amazing pain relief with this method. You can do this method at home. Instructions on how to do this appear later in the book. This method is great for causing a proliferation of fibroblasts (scar tissue producing cells) and fibroblast activity. Works extremely well for degenerative tendon issues.

- **Lymphatic Drainage**: Works great if you are older and have circulation issues. If you have any kind of nerve damage or long standing disorders in the legs, this therapy can help you a lot. If you have had severe edema for years, you should give this one a shot. This therapy should work alongside other therapies, and should not be depended on to fix the causes of your pain. This therapy speeds up metabolic waste exchange and will boost the effects of other therapies.

- **Taping:** Some injuries need lots of tape; others injuries, not so much. If I recommend it later on in the book for your injury, give it a try. To apply the tape properly requires practice, but if it is done right, you can get some major pain relief. Also keep in mind that you get what you pay for when it comes to athletic tape. Leukotape® and KT Tape® are recommended. If you buy cheap athletic tape from the drug store, you will have horrible results and you will be frustrated.

- **Chiropractic:** I love some chiropractic methods, and hate some as well. I recommend looking up reviews on individual chiropractors and finding the ones that consistently give people results. Some soft tissue injuries can benefit from chiropractic adjustment, but not all of them. They are great with nerve entrapment and bone alignment, but if that is not causing your issue, you usually do not have to see a chiropractor (in my opinion). Lots of chiropractors today are familiarizing themselves with soft tissue mobilization techniques. These chiropractors are great and give you amazing results; try to find these therapists as soon as you can. They have a good sense of how everything works together and can give you some great, long lasting results. To summarize: some chiropractors are miracle workers; some are a complete waste of time. Look up reviews and ask around your town to see who the best is.

- **Rolfing®:** Great postural mechanics therapy. This therapy deals with how fascia (connective tissue) can be manipulated and changed to better suite a person's activities. It also teaches you how to have better posture so that dysfunction has less reason to occur.

- **Physical Therapy:** I would not recommend it unless they are a special type of physical therapist that has certification in some form of soft tissue mobilization. Physical therapists love to make people stretch muscles with trigger points (making them worse and more painful), and love to try to strengthen regions of the body that have dysfunctional fascia (which leads to more pain). They do have an important place in the medical world when it comes to post surgery movement techniques and therapies. When it comes to chronic injuries, the results they give are slower than any of the previous therapies I have mentioned. They are very smart and have credentials, but they do not have the right protocols in place.

- **Cold Laser (or Low Level Laser Therapy®, LLLT®):** Some people love it, some people do not. If the issue you have is very superficial, then it would more than likely respond in your favor. There are no side effects and it is safer than anything though, it just costs quite a bit of money.

I would recommend going if the soft tissue mobilization methods I mentioned earlier failed to give results. The only thing you could really lose by trying this therapy is money.

- **Prolotherapy** ®: I love this therapy, but ONLY for certain injuries. This therapy works wonders for meniscus tears and other joint dysfunctions, but for other injuries, it does not seem to have as good of an effect. If I recommend Prolotherapy ® for an individual injury later in this book, it is worth your time. Some injuries need Prolotherapy ® to start the healing process again. You must go at least 4 times or more to see good results.

- **Voodoo Wrap**®: A great soft tissue mobilization method that uses a constricting band around an area of dysfunctional tissue to regain a more fluid and functional state. This method uses sheer force to break apart adhesions between fascia sheets, giving the area more nutrient exchange potential and much more. I like to use a bicycle inner tube because it is much cheaper and gives you the same results. All you have to do is cut open a bicycle tube lengthwise so that you end up with a long belt of rubber. Then, you wrap the tube around the area of dysfunction very tightly. Next, you move the joints that are associated with the area of dysfunction, and after 40-60 seconds of movement, you take the band off. You can do this over and over again and get some great results. This is also great to use if you have edema from an injury. It pushes the metabolic waste products out of the tissue and back into the veins and lymphatic system so that healing can take place much faster.

- **Myofascial Release**®: Can be hard to find a practitioner in your area. They work extremely well for really chronic injuries. If you have had issues for over a year, they will be able to give you some pretty amazing results. They are more patient then most therapists because of the prolonged duration of each treatment, and have a great deal of knowledge when it comes to how fascia works (especially its contractile properties). I would suggest going to this kind of therapist at least 3 times to see results.

- **Micro Current:** Works well for some nerve disorders, but I have not seen as good of results with chronic injuries. I have read so many articles about microcurrent, but all the machines I have used have not produced the results I have wanted. I know that people with fibromyalgia have benefited from this therapy greatly, especially when the practitioner has gloves on to administer treatment. Also, people with myofascial pain syndrome can get some good results as well. I would save my time and money though and try other therapies before trying this one.

- **Hot and Cold Treatments:** I used to be all for ice/heat treatments because everyone recommends it. I later found out that ice it isn't doing anything but lessening the pain, and heat speeds up metabolism, but not much else. It really does not fix any of the things that are causing the pain, and does not fix any of the perpetuating factors. I would not spend my time or money for the heating/icing products available today (some of which are extremely expensive). Usually what this therapy does is simply over stimulate sensory nerve receptors so that you do not feel as much pain. Who cares about numbing the pain when the causes are not addressed? We need pain, but we need to fix the cause of the pain.

- **TENS's Unit:** Only for dealing with the pain. All these machines do is over-stimulate the sensory nerve fibers of any area, which will result in fewer pain signals being perceived. It is nice to use if you have been in pain for months, but it isn't going to fix any of the causes of your pain. I have found that in a couple large muscle groups (such as the back and glutes), over stimulating a chronically contracted muscle can produce some benefit, but this is only for some muscles. I like to massage the electrodes into deep muscles with dysfunction, and when I hit a trigger point, I know it. The over excitement of muscle fibers in the trigger point cause it to contract so hard that it runs out of calcium, then it relaxes. This is not entirely proven to help, but like I said, in the glutes and back, it can seem to help without much risk. The machines are cheap and easily found online.

- **Orthopedic Doctor:** I find that they have their purpose in severe or traumatic physical injuries. They do a great job of fixing things that were recently broken in the body. When it comes to chronic and degenerative pain issues, they are horrible. Most chronic natured injuries do not respond very well to surgery. The reason why is because most of the surgeries are simply trying to get rid of excess scar tissue or to get rid of the broken pieces (such as in a meniscectomy or plantar fascia release). These surgeries have lots of implications and complications. The rest after the surgery can cause many of issues, and the surgery itself is quite a bit of trauma on its own. Some argue in the literature that the positive results of these surgeries come from the actual rest the person is forced to experience after the surgery. People do not like to rest unless they are forced to. Sometimes the person just needs to rest the area (without surgery), then fix the dysfunctional tissue around the injury, then they are good to go (and with a lot more money in their pocket!). However, it is always smart to check with an orthopedic doctor so that you can get a clear diagnosis of your condition. If you have extreme damage, you may be a good candidate for surgery.

- **Cupping Therapy/Gua Sha:** These are great for breaking up adhesions in the fascial system. The only problem I see with these adhesion release therapies as compared to other ones is that they are overdone. Gua Sha treatments should not cause excessive bruising. Also, cupping therapy should not be left on for 30 minutes at a time, which causes black bruises. Having a light pressure gua sha treatment or cupping treatment works fine. You can also buy these tools online and teach yourself how to do it in about ten minutes. They are super easy to use and cost effective if you buy your own tools. They also are said to help with lymphatic drainage. They do cause lymphatic drainage, but not nearly as effectively or systematically as actual lymphatic drainage therapies.

How to Progress with MSTR Therapy

This guide will discuss how quickly you should move through my program. The speed at which you move through the program depends heavily on how much damage is inflicted on your body. Each person's body and pain is different, so be sure to start slow and progress consistently over time through each step of my program.

1. Fix your diet now (next chapter). You need a good solid diet because your diet is your foundation. If you have a bad diet, you cannot expect any of these therapies to work at their full potential. If you have a good diet, your pain will improve and the results from the therapies you are currently doing will work faster and give more pain relief than you can imagine.

2. If you need to tape for your injury, start now. The sooner you start the better. I list some recommendations in the individual injuries section, but looking up taping methods online is smarter because there are so many ways to tape for every injury out there. Some people respond to different taping techniques, so it is smart to try them all to see what works for your injury.

3. MSTR:

    *   Release the trigger points and do fascia adhesion scraping around twice a day for about two weeks. After the trigger points are released and the fascia is unrestricted, you will have a new understanding of what is causing your pain and how you can fix it yourself. When you feel comfortable with first two steps, you are ready to move on. Your muscles and ligaments will feel different and your pain should decrease. This is when you know you are ready to stretch.

    *   Follow the kinetic chain stretches as outlined for your injury. Do these once a day along with the trigger point methods and scraping. If you feel that the trigger points are gone and the muscles feel nice and soft and do not have any connective tissue adhesions, you can stop those therapies and stick with just the kinetic chain stretches.

4. Follow any additional therapies that I recommend for your injury during or after MSTR.

As you have probably noticed, MSTR is composed of 3 major steps if it is to be used as a therapeutic tool to give consistent results. The order of MSTR is extremely important; if done in the right order, MSTR will invoke serious amounts of pain relief. Here is a quick summary of the functional steps of MSTR:

- **Trigger Point Therapy**: Fix muscle dysfunction by applying a <u>blunt stroking pressure</u> to a muscle that is <u>relaxed</u> and <u>shortened</u>.

- **Fascia Adhesion Release Therapy**: Fix fascia dysfunction by <u>scraping an aggressive and angled pressure</u> to a dysfunctional area of fascia while the fascia and/or muscle unit is <u>relaxed</u> and <u>stretched</u>.

- **Kinetic Chain Stretch Therapy**: Fixes the long-term causes of joint/muscle/fascia dysfunction dynamics so that problem does not come back. These stretches cannot be done until AFTER trigger points and fascia adhesions are resolved. These stretches are done by putting <u>multiple joints in a kinetic chain in a static stretch</u>, all at the same time. These stretches must keep all joints involved within a healthy range of motion (unlike conventional stretching which puts joints into unstable and dangerous positions). During this kind of stretch, the <u>muscles composing the kinetic chain must be released</u> (usually by flexing an opposing muscle group) <u>so that instead of stretching muscle, we stretch the dysfunctional sheets of fascia which lie between and around the muscles</u>.

This book has a huge "muscle guide" that shows all the muscles that tend to become dysfunctional, where the trigger points are (shown with big X's), and where the fascia adhesions like to be (shown in circle areas). I will first go over how to actually do the trigger point therapy/fascia adhesion release through scraping/kinetic chain stretches, and then you will use the muscle guide to find out where the trigger points and fascia adhesions are for your particular injury. After you take care of the trigger points and fascia adhesions, you can move on to the section on kinetic chain stretches. It usually takes 2-3 weeks to take care of the trigger points/dysfunctional fascia adhesions, but can take less or more time depending on your injury.

When you should NOT use MSTR

MSTR is made for chronic inflammatory injuries that can't seem to go away. It does not work for all kinds of pain. Here is the list of diseases/disorders/implications to MSTR:

1. If you're obese. Fix your weight with the "Chronic Pain Diet" ahead then come back to MSTR. It is really hard to invoke changes on the body if you have lots of fatty tissues in the way. If you have an ankle/knee issue, you can still use MSTR. But for most other injuries, you're going to have to lose the weight first. Losing weight is not about working out. Working out can be dangerous. Instead, make your diet absolutely perfect and the weight will fall right off.

2. You have an obvious bone fracture. You need to see an orthopedic doctor now.

3. You have bone cancer.

4. You are pregnant.

5. You have severe arthritis or an inflammatory disease. Try my chronic pain diet first, and if the pain improves with diet alone, and you are more functional, give MSTR a shot. But be very careful and go slowly!

6. You have had a recent injury to Muscle/Bones/Fascia/Cartilage etc. MSTR is for those stubborn chronic pain injuries that like to stay around for years, or that last bit of pain that just won't leave. Also, MSTR is also aimed at fixing the causes of your pain, so wait until the injury heals all the way, and then find out what caused the pain, and fix that.

    If you have had a recent injury, rest the area and let pain guide you on what you should and should not do. Drink plenty of water and make your diet perfect. If the pain is around for 4, 6, or even 8 weeks, time to start MSTR. If you start MSTR with a recent injury that is not healed, you will cause more damage. You can always go to an Active Release Technique ® therapist or Rolfing ® therapist to see what they can do if you are desperate. Orthopedic doctors are horrible when it comes to chronic injuries, but a lot of them are really great at fixing recent injuries. You may need to see an orthopedist for your injury and consider their advice.

MSTR: What happens when it does not work? How is this possible?

Every person is different. We develop and grow in interesting ways which gives way to a huge variety of bone structures, muscle strength and so much more. When you are trying to treat yourself or others with MSTR, you must keep this in mind. You must understand that what seems to work for everyone may not work for some people. I do believe that if you do **not** get pain relief with your efforts, you are looking in the wrong places. The body is very mechanical and nearly every kind of disorder in the body has an actual cause.

Do not feel frustrated when treatments do not give you results. It only means that you are overlooking the actual cause of the problem, you are not looking at the right organ systems, etc.

For example, just because you have lower back pain does not mean it is caused by a lower back muscle spasm. There are many other disorders that need to be ruled out if you are experiencing back pain. Be sure to go to a doctor that can evaluate you in person. I understand that it can be expensive, but they will give you an opinion that can save you a lot of time and grief. If you go from doctor to doctor, and they all seemed to rule out other disorders, then give this book a solid shot. Do everything in the proper order and see what your results are.

This book lays out protocols for care for each and every major area of the body (and common ailments). Protocols are unfortunately never perfect, but they are a good start. When you are finished reading this book, you might even be able to make your own methods. This is because once you understand the organ systems inflicted in chronic inflammatory injuries, and how they work, you will be able to know how to fix them. You will come up with new treatment methods on the fly and be able to find makeshift tools everywhere.

This book is here to give you the concept of fixing chronic inflammatory injuries. It will be your job to make your own style of use. Many of these methods can be changed or modified to suite a specific person. Some people are big, some are small. Some are round, some are thin. You must take this all into consideration when you are working on someone's body (or your own body). Just because foam rolling works for my small stature body, does not mean it will work for everyone. Just remember the basics to MSTR and you will be able to make your own treatments with your own tools.

If you or a client you have been seeing does not experience amazing results with my methods, you are probably looking in the wrong place. Maybe it is a hormone issue that is causing the problem. Maybe it is a nerve disorder. Maybe they have a rare disorder that a previous doctor overlooked. You must keep this in mind at all times. These methods are made to fix chronic inflammatory injuries. If you do not get fast results from these methods, you most likely have something else that is causing the pain.

The First Foundational Step

To Pain Free Living: Diet

If you want the MSTR to fix your pain, you need to fix your diet first. The foods that you eat can influence hormone levels, systematic healing capacity, nerve firing rates and many other physiological changes in the body that directly or indirectly cause people more or less pain (or perpetuate current pain levels).

The average American diet is filled with foods that cause havoc on the body. When you combine the average American diet with a chronic injury or any kind of chronic inflammation, the body has no choice but to increase the pain levels. The foods you eat dictate how your body will perform. The human body is a robust structure in many ways, but if you do not give it the proper building blocks, it will fall apart, sometimes quite literally.

The body simply responds to what is given to it. We are what we eat. If you eat pain provoking foods, you will have more pain than if you did not have them.

One thing that people truly need to understand is that there are no "silver bullets" that will instantly make you healthy. You cannot just expect any single pill to fix your health, or have the expectation that seeing your doctors/therapist will instantly "cure" you on the spot.

Regardless of what surgery you get, how much MSTR you do to yourself daily, and how much money you have, it all does not matter if your diet is weak. Having a weak diet causes your body to work extra hard to sustain itself. If you have a well-planned diet for pain, other therapies you are currently undertaking will have boosted favorable effects. If you are not seeing results with the current therapies you are on, maybe your diet is the weakest link causing you not to see favorable results.

You cannot eat fast food every day for a month, then "clean out the toxins" in one afternoon with some "toxin cleanse" that you read in a magazine. What is needed is a complete diet change to provoke nearly permanent results in the reduction of your pain levels. A lot of people that try my diet usually notice that their skin looks better, they have more energy, and when they see these results, it is extremely hard to let go of the diet. It is hard for most people to change to the diet in this book at first, but once you start seeing results from it, you will never want to go back.

Chronic and Systemic Inflammation

Can Be Changed With Diet

If you are in pain, you have inflammation. If you have had pain for more than 6-8 weeks, it is chronic inflammation. Inflammation is a healthy and normal response to handle trauma and damage inflicted to the body. It is also used in response to infections. You need inflammation, or you would be dead. If you did not have inflammation, you would not be able to repair injuries as fast, and your immune system would be compromised.

What we do not want is chronic inflammation. Chronic inflammation is "bad inflammation". When chronic inflammation sets in, the body gives up on healing all together. After 6 weeks of inflammation, the area starts to become "degenerative". The body starts breaking the area down because it has "given up" on fixing it. We do not want this. We want inflammation, but we do not want chronic inflammation.

The foods you eat influence the chemicals made in your body. Some foods that you eat encourage chronic inflammation promoting chemicals. They cause the chronic inflammation to set in faster, and for longer. If you eat foods that encourage chronic inflammation, it makes it extremely hard to heal from injuries.

When your entire diet is filled with foods that encourage chronic inflammation, a different beast comes to wreak havoc. It goes by the name of "systemic inflammation". What this means is that the entire body is in a state of "mild" inflammation. This hinders your body's healing performance greatly. It also takes a lot of energy to sustain this systemic inflammation response.

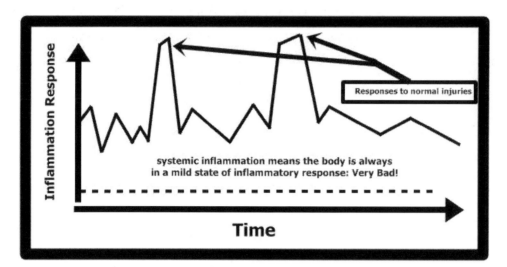

Unhealthy and Chronic Inflammation Response Example

What we want to do is change the diet so that the body produces chemicals that stop chronic inflammation and systemic inflammation. These responses are bad. They degrade the body, use tons of energy, and do not help anything. But we need inflammation in order to heal. The diet that you need to have instead is one that encourages a healthy inflammatory response. Here is an example of what your inflammation response would look like with the right kind of diet:

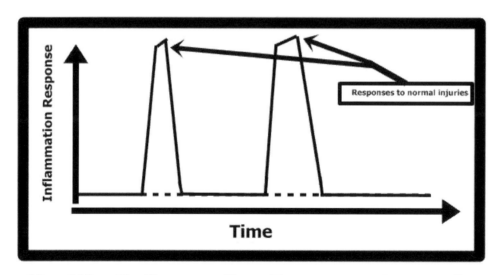

Healthy Inflammation Response Example

Notice in the picture above how the body has no inflammation most of the time, and then the spikes indicate an inflammation response to fix an injury (or infection). This is healthy. The food you choose to eat can either help you have healthy inflammation responses, or can cause you to have chronic/systemic inflammation responses. When you have chronic/systemic inflammation, you are always in pain, and the injuries you have seem to never heal. When you have healthy inflammation responses, the body fixes what it needs to, and then moves on.

Will a good diet fix my pain completely?

For some people it will. Results vary. For me, I need this diet in order to walk. I cannot walk if I eat foods that promote inflammation (And this happens within hours. Part of my nerve disorder is that the effects are instant).

If you have a chronic tendon injury, I would expect at least a 20%-35% change in pain levels. For some people, this diet will fix their pain greatly. For others, it will only reduce the pain. I am pretty confident of my diet because I have experimented on myself and others in pain for over 4 years, and have a good feel for what really works and what does not.

Having this diet in combination with other treatments is the best option. The diet is the foundation, and you build on that with MSTR and other therapy options.

Is this a temporary diet?

No. It is a lifestyle that you need to stick with. If you do not like pain, and do not want it to come back, you need to make this diet a part of your life and stick with it 100%. After your pain is gone, an organic paleo diet is most ideal. This prevents systemic inflammation and gives you a strong body. I have found that paleo diet does not help much when you are in pain, unfortunately.

I would be very cautious when others try to tell you what to eat. Some examples of people that you should NOT listen to:

- Obese/unhealthy looking doctors. I once saw one of my doctors eating Doritos and soda at the movie theater. The next day I heard him tell a lady in his office "you should not have any soda; it is horrible for your bones". He is also obese. You should not listen to doctors that do not practice what they preach. Look for a healthy and robust looking doctor. Look at their skin, look at their build. You can learn a lot about someone's health from just looking at them. Find doctors that give you a good example to follow.

- People that are not in chronic pain, or do not understand how it functions. Your friends and family may think that they can help your pain with their dietary suggestions. Usually this information is far from being correct and needs to be ignored. Disregard information from these people.

I am personally tired of seeing physical education teachers at schools that are unhealthier than the kids they coach (most, if not all, of my P.E. teachers in high school/college were obese and had health problems).

I do not understand it when I see a doctor/nurse smoking cigarettes, then a few minutes later tell their patients not to smoke. I like doctors/nurses that stand by the advice they give.

A lot of the health advice out there is based off of medical studies that are funded by companies that do not care about YOUR health and are just trying to sell you their products. Be wary of these studies.

Then what makes a diet "Perfect" for reducing pain?
The best diets for pain are the ones that are done through trial and error, and with the individual in mind. There is not a single diet that is "perfect" for anyone simply because everyone needs different amounts of nutrients at different times of day. Keep trying new variations of foods in the "food list" ahead to find out what works best with your body.

Positive thinking and hope can only get you so far
The body responds to what you give it. It is a machine that works well if you give it what it needs. Positive thinking and hope does not help change your diet. What you need to do is make this new diet a part of your life, and stick with it 100%. Also, the change into this diet should be fast. Making slow changes every day does not help your pain now. If you want to help relieve the pain, do the diet now. Your diet is your foundation. You are in a sense "what you eat" and nothing more. Give your body the food it needs to be healthy and it will thank you by reducing your pain and speeding up your healing abilities.

Most of the diet is based off of raw foods. Why raw foods?
Raw foods have enzymes, and cooked foods do not because heat destroys enzymes. When you eat cooked foods, you need to break it down to its rudimentary parts so that it can be assimilated by the body. Enzymes are needed to break down the cooked food so that it can be used by the body. It cannot be used by the body if enzymes are not present during digestion. We can make enzymes on our own, but it takes a lot of "grunt" work. Enzymes for digestion of cooked foods are made by the pancreas. These enzymes are complex protein structures that take a lot of energy to create - energy that could be better used for repairing damage in the body and other more important bodily functions.

"Cooked food" that does not get completely digested (due to the lack of enzymes or other factors) makes its way into the body (by way of the blood stream) as a "circulating immune complex" (CIC), which in turn has to be removed from the body by the immune system (broken down by macrophages [cells that clean the blood], as this undigested food is seen as a "foreign invader" in the body). The process to get these CICs out of the body is inflammation. This is a full body inflammatory reaction and is a form of systemic inflammation. Long story short, cooked food is BAD!

Raw foods have all the enzymes intact and are ready to break down the nutrients in the food (cooked foods have zero enzymes because heat destroys enzymes). When you eat enzyme-rich raw foods, you get tons of nutrients that your body can use. The nutrients that are in cooked foods are still there, but you cannot use them until your body makes the enzymes to digest it. As said earlier, this takes a lot of energy. The nutrients in the cooked food are also degraded. Vitamins and other nutrients are extremely heat sensitive. When you cook food, not only do you kill all of the enzymes, you also destroy vitamins and nutrients. It also makes the oils in the food rancid, which can lead to other problems. Rancid oils are not helpful; raw oils are.

Cooked Foods=No Enzymes= More Pain!

Can I have a cheat meal? Can I have "moderation" of junk food?
Never! This should not cross your mind. If you want more pain, have a cheat meal. If you do not like pain, do not have a cheat meal ever.

Moderation does not work. Going 99% of the way will not give you the pain relief you truly want. Think of junk food as an addiction similar to drug addiction. If you have drugs once a month, you are still hurting yourself. Junk food cannot be in moderation; it should be removed completely and forever. Think only of what you can eat, then ignore everything else. This will give you a new life with less pain.

Eating healthy is extremely fun, and makes you feel amazing! It can be hard at first to make the change, but do it. Do it now and forever.

A Note on chewing
When you spend extra time to chew your food up all the way, it makes it easier for the enzymes to do their job at breaking the food down into the nutrients/vitamins/minerals that you so desperately need. Chewed food has more surface area for the enzymes to attach to. This means that the more chewed the food is, the more digested and usable the food becomes.

Drink good sourced water!

Municipal tap water is not good for you. Buy a quality filter, or buy natural spring water from the store. Avoid tap water. Also, try to drink more water than you think you need. Carry a water bottle around and drink out of it often. Whenever you have inflammation, the body has to carry a plethora of wastes out of the body. One way it does this is by using the kidneys to filter the wastes from the blood. The blood carries a lot of the wastes that are produced by the chemical reactions from inflammation. What is also in this blood is water. When you drink excess water, your body has to remove it from the body. When the water is being removed from the blood via the kidneys, the inflammation wastes are removed with the water. More water = faster removal of inflammatory waste products = faster healing.

Long story short, drink clean water, and very often. You will be peeing a lot, but it will be worth the effort. I would say that 35% of the results of your diet will be from how much water you drink. Drink it often. I do not count how many "glasses" of water I drink, I simply drink water all the time, and so should you.

What makes a food anti-inflammatory?

First, none of the foods in my program stop inflammation entirely. They stop chronic/systematic inflammation. We still need healthy forms of inflammation. The foods in this program do just that. They contain certain chemical compounds that cause the body to produce other chemicals that promote good inflammation. Other "bad foods" that we are avoiding in this program contain chemicals that make the inflammation worse by promoting systemic/chronic inflammation. I will refrain from listing the bad foods in the diet program, because there are millions of them. Processed foods of all kinds will not be on the list. You need whole raw food if you want pain relief. Stick to the list of foods I will show you, and you will be good to go.

How often should I eat?

As often as you can, but in very small meals (or snacks). Three meals a day causes your hormone levels to go berserk after you eat, causing changes in the body that are unwanted by someone in pain. I find that snacking throughout the day is the best way to reduce pain and still get plenty of nutrients. Schedules are hard to follow, and can cause stress. What has given me the best results is to eat a couple bites every half an hour, and skip the whole "meal time" regime entirely.

I bring food with me, in my car and everywhere I go so that I can always snack. It is not hard to bring the food along. You do not need to prepare the foods because they are raw. Stick a carrot in a bag, bring it with you and then eat it when you get hungry. This is very easy to do and requires no preparation at all.

Prescription drugs and Nsaids

I understand that some prescription drugs that you take need to be taken to keep you alive. What you do not want to do is take them without knowing how they work in the body. Read as much as you can about the drugs you are on so you can see what they are doing in your body. Usually, they fight for absorption with other vitamins and minerals that your body needs. It is best to read about what vitamins and minerals you are at risk for being deficient in from taking your prescription medications, and taking said vitamins/minerals on alongside the diet.

I am on an anti-convulsant for my nerve disorder. I have no choice but to take it; otherwise, my walking abilities would be reduced to half the distance I can walk right now. It does compete for absorption with calcium and vitamin D. I take calcium and vitamin D on the side. I watch my blood levels and get bone density scans to gauge my results to be sure that I am good to go.

This is very simple "preventative maintenance" that everyone should be doing so that they can save themselves from future pain. The last thing you want when you're in pain is more injuries. Usually when one thing in the body breaks, other things will to follow suit.

NSAIDS (Non Steroidal Anti-Inflammatory Drugs) Cause the body to cease inflammation processes in the body. What happens when the body does not have inflammation is horrible. Wastes accumulate, and healing takes place very slowly. We cannot have this. I understand that a lot of people take these anti inflammatory drugs for pain, but understand that they have many hazardous side effects on the body. Usually pain is good to have, so you can understand what parts of your body need attention. When you stop this pain signal from happening, you go on to further hurt the injury and you never become better. You need pain. If you ignore it, your health will get worst and the pain will stay with you for much longer.

The better choice instead of NSAIDS is to give the body the nutrients it needs to speed up healing and provide you with a strong and powerful inflammatory response that can fix the problems causing you pain.

What can Vitamin/Mineral/Enzyme/Herb Supplements do for my pain?

There are a lot of supplements out there that can seriously help reduce your pain. My favorite kind, by far, has to be systematic enzymes. These are super effective and help your body to fix old injuries and literally stop the chemicals in your body that are causing you to have chronic/systemic inflammation. These enzymes are extremely safe and you can take them every day for the rest of your life without any side effects.

Some mineral supplements are a good idea to take because modern food does not have many minerals in them. The soil where most of our food comes from is over farmed and deprived of the nutrients we need from it. Two mineral supplements, Magnesium and MSM, are practically required to be taken if you are in pain. These two supplements used to be abundant in the soil many years ago, but are now present in minuscule amounts. It is better and cheaper just to take these supplements in addition to the diet.

Some vitamins are just needed when you're in pain, such as vitamin D. There are many benefits that will be listed later.

Herbs are great. Different herbs promote production of certain chemicals that help rid your body of the bad inflammation. The hard part is finding good sources for your herbs. Always try to by organic and locally grown herbs.

What is next?
Let's move on to the "food list". Remember; only consume what is on the list, and nothing else.

Bring the list with you everywhere. Photocopy it or write it down on paper, and make sure you have it present every time you want to eat.

The Food List

Think of these foods as medicine for pain.

Vegetables

- Arugula
- Asparagus
- Avocado
- Beets
- Broccoli
- Capers
- Cauliflower
- Crookneck squash
- Cucumbers
- Fennel bulb
- Horseradish
- Leek
- Lettuce (butter, endive, radicchio, baby spring mix)
- Kale
- Mushrooms
- Mustard greens
- Onions
- Spinach
- Swiss chard
- Watercress

Sprouts

- Alfalfa
- Broccoli
- Buckwheat
- Mung Bean
- Red clover
- Fenugreek
- Mustard seed
- Wheat Grass
- Sunflower

Berries

- Bilberry
- Blackberry
- Boysenberry
- Cranberry
- Hawthorne berry
- Juniper berry
- Loganberry
- Mulberry
- Raspberry
- Red currant
- Strawberry

Fruits

- Apricot
- Cherries
- Coconut
- Figs
- Guava
- Honeydew melon
- Kiwi
- Lemon
- Lime
- Mandarin orange
- Nectarine
- Olives
- Papaya
- Passion fruit
- Peach
- Pear
- Persimmon
- Pineapple
- Plum
- Pomegranate (Raw only, not the juice they sell in stores!)
- Star fruit
- Tangerine
- Rhubarb

Herbs / Spices

- Allspice
- Anise
- Basil
- Bay leaf
- Cayenne
- Chamomile
- Chives
- Cilantro
- Cinnamon
- Cloves
- Cumin
- Dill
- Elephant garlic
- Fenugreek
- Ginger
- Hawthorne leaf

- Marigold flowers
- Marjoram
- Mustard (seed, leaf)
- Noni
- Nutmeg
- Oregano
- Paprika
- Peppermint
- Rosemary
- Sage
- Spearmint
- Tarragon
- Thyme
- Turmeric
- Vanilla bean
- Yucca

Miscellaneous

- Nutritional Yeast Flakes
- Sauerkraut (Only Raw. Most on the market are not)
- Spirulina
- Pickled Vegetables
- Apple Cider Vinegar
- Fresh/Raw Wheat Grass Juice

Natural Sweeteners

- Stevia

Nuts and Seeds

- Almonds
- Sunflower seeds
- Flaxseed
- Pumpkin seeds
- Brazil nuts
- Anise seed
- Pine nuts
- Cashews
- Fennel seed
- Caraway seed
- Sesame seeds

Protein Sources

- Almonds
- Avocado
- Mushrooms
- Sprouts
- Pumpkin Seeds
- Sprouts

Great Fatty Acid Oils (Must be Extra Virgin/Cold Pressed)

- Avocado Oil
- Apricot Kernel Oil
- Almond Oil
- Flaxseed Oil
- Olive Oil
- Hazelnut Oil

Medicinal Herbs

- Angelica
- Aloe
- Ashwagandha
- Black Cohosh
- Devils Claw
- Fever Few
- Turmeric (1st Favorite)
- Boswellia (2nd Favorite)
- White Poplar
- White Willow Bark (3rd Favorite)
- Winter Green
- Wormwood

Food Proportion Amounts

One thing that we must understand is that everyone's body needs different amounts of individual nutrients. This pie chart should give you an idea of how much of each kind of food group to eat, but you will need to experiment with different proportion sizes of each food group to see what works for you. It is really safe to experiment with proportion sizes of all food groups except for fruit.

Fruit is the only food group that you can easily "over indulge" if you are in pain, and can easily cause more pain if you have too much. Fruit is very healthy, but with small amounts. It is also best to eat fruit by itself. All of the other food groups can be eaten together at any time. Two kinds of fruit that can be eaten all the time and without much moderation are avocado and coconut.

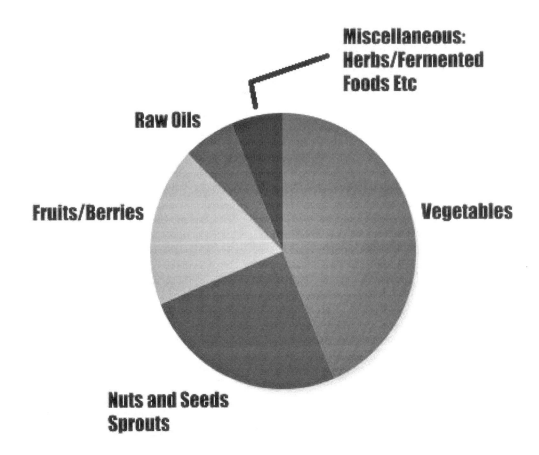

I do not like vegetables... Can I avoid them?

No. You need them. I hear a lot of people complain about eating raw vegetables when I give them my food list, and I tell them very nicely that they have to "deal with it".

You must understand that when you become an adult you have to do a lot of things that you do not want to do. Such as, doing the dishes, paying bills, and now, eating vegetables. Do not eat for enjoyment; eat for good health. Get your enjoyment later from not being in pain. Would you rather be in pain 24/7 and enjoying the foods you eat for 1 hour of that day, or instead, feeling great 24/7 and eating only for health? When your body adapts to the increase in vegetables, you'll start to love them. Vegetables are required if you want this program to be successful for you.

Why aren't dairy products on the list? How will I get my calcium if I cannot have dairy products?

No human being should consume dairy products. Dairy is designed to sustain a baby cow, or calf. Calves use their mother's milk to gain substantial amounts of weight after they are born. It should not be in your body. When you drink it, you are being introduced to chemicals that make your hormones go crazy. (The calf has different hormone needs than you do. When you drink cow's milk, your body responds to those chemicals present in the milk that were made for the calf. You do not want this. It also is filled with sugar and too much protein, without any fiber. When you have too much sugar without fiber, you get a super high insulin spike, which is not good for pain. Also, when you have too much protein without fiber, your body flushes it out through the kidneys. Problem is, when your body flushes protein from the kidneys, it also leeches out calcium with it.

There are tons of studies in the medical literature today that say dairy products do not help osteoporosis. Remember, this substance is for calves. You may ask "what about cheese?" and the answer is still a big no. On top of not being healthy, cheese is more processed than milk. Even if it is raw milk or raw cheese, do not eat it. Processed or not, you do not need these things in your body.

The good news is, there are tons of plants that have loads of usable calcium. Remember, cows only eat grass, yet they are making calcium rich milk out of the grass they eat, all day long.

Vegetables have tons of calcium. Stick to the food list and your calcium needs will be fulfilled.

Are fruit juices and dried fruit ok?

Think of these two items as pure sugar. Sugar is horrible when you are in pain. Fruit juices that are bought from the store are cooked before they reach the store shelves. This means that all those "life giving" and "pain relieving" enzymes are not present in the juice. Also, the heat changes the structure of the sugars in the fruit juices. When you cook the fruit sugars, they are not the same. They are degraded in ways that are unfavorable for the body. The enzymes, vitamins, and minerals are changed, and this is horrible for your pain levels. Your body needs fruits how they came from nature, fresh and raw.

Dried fruit is pretty much the same as eating candy. You do not want this in your body. Even common dried fruits such as raisins should be avoided completely.

If you want to make your own "fresh and raw" juices, go right on ahead, BUT you must mix the pulp and the juice together after you are done juicing it. In order to use the enzymes, you need to drink the juice/pulp mixture as soon as you can after it is made. Oxidization loves to set in after you make fresh/raw juice, so be sure to drink it fast! Also, fruit juices/pulp has to be used very sparingly; but, you can have as much vegetable juice/pulp as you would like.

Some great juice/pulp combinations are: Beets, carrot, sprouted almonds, cucumber, pear, spinach and pineapple. These are extremely enzyme rich (especially the beets and pineapple), and great to add to your diet in a juice/pulp concoction.

No more Alcohol/Drugs/Cigarettes/Coffee/Caffeine of any kind
These seem to be commonplace in the American lifestyle. These substances only cause harm to the body, and literally create and exacerbate pain in many ways. It is best to just avoid them completely. Do not have "a little bit" of any of these substances. Alcohol, Drugs, and Cigarettes need to be stopped if you are in pain, or if you care any bit about your health. There are millions of reasons to stop, and tons of great resources on how to get over the addiction. Make it your life's goal to stop these habits right now and forever.

Caffeine is a type of drug. It is addictive and not healthy for you at all. Caffeine perpetuates trigger points (these cause lots of pain in the muscle system of the body) and stimulates the nerve system in ways that are extremely unfavorable for someone in pain. These habits should be stopped completely if you want reduction in pain levels. I understand that to avoid withdrawal symptoms, you must stop consuming caffeine gradually. This does not mean over the course of months. This means that you should stop within a week or so. You can "gradually" quit in two weeks.

What about my "healthy" and organic/natural herbal teas that contain a tiny bit of caffeine?

These should not be taken, even in small doses. They are wreaking havoc on your body. If it has caffeine at all, do not drink it. With that said, there are tons of great herbal teas that taste amazing and are completely caffeine free! Do not use honey or any other kind of sugar to sweeten your tea, ever. Use stevia. Even a small amount of honey is unfavorable to someone in pain. Avoid it at all costs.

What about Agave Nectar/Coconut Sugar/Honey and all of the other sweeteners on the market?

You do not need them. They are not helping you. Even if they are low on the "glycemic index" (which is indeed important), they are still a huge carbohydrate load that your body does not need. It is best to get your carbohydrates from other sources that are more pure, such as raw fruit. Even then, you do not want to have an overload of fruit. Sugar can cause pain if you have enough of it in your system regardless of where it came from.

Why are Tomatoes/Eggplant/Most kinds of potatoes/Okra/Most Peppers not on the list??

They belong to the dangerous nightshade family of plants. They contain molecular compounds that promote inflammation soon after eating them. These should be avoided at all costs. The effects of nightshade plants alone can cause someone extreme amounts of pain and promotes chronic/systematic inflammation processes. Take them out of your life and avoid them completely.

Why should I eat sprouts? Can I eat raw nuts and seeds?

Sprouts are extremely healthy to eat. These little wonders of plant life have so many nutrients and enzymes, it is mind boggling. They are filled with complete proteins and important fatty acids. They are also extremely filling and should be one of the main "staples" of your pain diet.

When plants release nuts and seeds into the environment, they expect animals to eat them. When a raw seed or nut is eaten by an animal (like a human), it goes through the digestive system of the animal pretty easily and unharmed. It is then pooped out of the animal, and the nut or seed is at an advantage because it is in a pile of fertilizer (the animal's poop). I am sure many of you reading this have seen sunflower seeds pass through their digestive system, and into the toilet with no problems. Why is this so? Why did the enzymes not break it down? It is because raw nuts and seeds contain enzyme inhibitors. These make it nearly impossible for us to digest it, even if we chew it up. The enzyme inhibitors will still be there no matter how hard we chew, and we lose all the chances to assimilate the nutrients in the nut or seed.

I get it, great poop story, but how do I make it easier to digest these seeds? By germinating them. This is the "first step" in sprouting. All you do is take the nuts or seeds you want to eat and properly digest, and let them soak in water for 8-12 hours. Rinse the seeds out in cold water. Bam, no more enzyme inhibitors! The soaking action of water causes the nuts and seeds to think that they are in a favorable environment to sprout. They think that they have already passed through the animal's digestive system, and it is time to grow into a big and strong plant. But they are wrong. We tricked the nuts and seeds, and we can now eat them and digest them easily.

Check out the "sprouts" list to learn about other nuts and seeds you can germinate. Germinating a nut or seed is the first step. If you continue growing the nut or seed, then it is considered a sprout. If you let it grow and develop until it requires sunlight (turns green and requires soil and more to grow), then it is considered a "micro green". Sprouts and micro greens are extremely healthy and filled with nutrients; try to get as much of these into your diet as possible.

The importance of fat in the diet and why you should eat raw oils only
You need fat. It is beyond the scope and practicality of this book, but understand that you need fat for millions of chemical processes in your body. With the proper choice of oils, you will have reduced pain. Fats are a crucial nutrient that has to be present in the body in order to have the body working efficiently.

What kinds of fats should I consume?
Raw fats. Raw oils. Why?

When you cook a fat, you make it rancid. You chemically degrade it. It changes into forms that it was not like before you cooked it. These are horrible things and bad for your health in so many ways. They promote systematic inflammation and extreme amounts of "oxidative stress" (exactly opposite to the positive effects of anti-oxidants). These unstable "cooked oils" should not be in the body of someone in pain.

I suggest a huge list of oils. When you buy them, they should say "cold pressed" and "extra virgin" or "raw" no matter what. If it does not say these words, do not buy it.

If you cook an oil or fat, it kills all the benefits. Do not eat cooked oils.

For example: If you want to eat coconut oil, take a spoon, scoop out a bit of coconut oil from your "raw coconut oil" jar, and eat it. If you want to eat some olive oil, sprinkle it on your vegetables. Just eat it. Never cook it. This simple habit should be made from now until forever. Eating the meat of a coconut has tons of rich fats that can help anyone. Also, lots of raw nuts and seeds have great fats, especially walnuts and almonds. (Try to always sprout these so you can digest them.)

Is this the perfect diet?

No. This diet strives to give you pain relief by fulfilling your bodies nutrient needs and reducing the junk that it does not need. The truth of the matter is that your body is always changing its needs. When you break a bone, you need more calcium. If you get a huge burn, your body is going to need more skin building blocks to repair the damage. Your body always needs different amounts of nutrients minute by minute, and even though this diet tries to give your body the perfect amounts of nutrients, you need to figure out what your body responds to best. Try every item on the food list, and find out what works best for you. The best combination in my opinion would be to have a single bite from everything on the list, every single day. This is obviously not very realistic, but should be what you are shooting for.

Is this diet ideal for following for the rest of my life?

I find that for a healthy individual, an organic Paleo diet without grains and with fresh fruits, vegetables and meats is the best. But for someone in pain, it just seems to make matters worse. I like to think that having a Paleo diet helps, but time and time again I find that the addition of meat causes excess pain. This may not be for all, especially if you have a small amount of pain, but if your pain is excessively chronic, my diet suggestions in this book should give you some of the best results ever compared to otherwise. If your pain is gone for a few months, and you are feeling great, you can slowly add some fish back in, then maybe some other meats, as long as they are organic and come from a local farm (ideally).

Vitamins, Minerals and Supplements for Pain

These vitamins and supplements should not be depended on to fix your pain alone. They need to be used synergistically with the diet. When these vitamins and supplements are combined with this diet, you will notice some big improvements. I also do not like vitamins and supplements that do not work. You need to be able to "feel" the results. Everything on this list is going to give you results if you combine it with a good diet. Be sure to read through each consideration for the vitamins and supplements mentioned below before you try them.

Systemic Enzymes

These are as close to a "magic potion" as you can get nowadays. These enzymes are specially formulated to give your body exactly what it needs when you are in chronic pain. They go through the blood stream and change the physiological environment in the body to improve healing. My favorite "general use" systemic enzyme is Wobenzym N ©. This product has never failed to deliver me results, and every time I refer people to using this stuff, they see results. It is great to use after surgeries or trauma of any kind. The benefits of systemic enzymes are widespread and beyond the scope of this book. These enzymes are used in Germany as a replacement for NSAIDS and give you results that you can actually FEEL. If you have inflammation, you should take systemic enzymes.

Some systemic enzymes, such as serrapeptase, have very interesting properties. This enzyme in particular can digest scar tissue. It literally goes into your blood and breaks apart scar tissue adhesions in various places in the body where scar tissue is present. This one is great to take after a huge surgery that involves lots of possible scarring.

How to take Systemic Enzymes

The number one thing you need to know about taking systemic enzymes is the fact that you MUST take them on an empty stomach. Then, you must wait an hour until you can eat again. They need to be on their own in the digestive system so they make it into your blood stream. If you take them with food, they will just digest the food present around the enzymes, and be "denatured" in a sense. A great time to take systemic enzymes is right when you wake up in the morning and right when you go to bed. Be sure to wait at least an hour after taking them before eating your first meal or snack. Be sure to also have your last meal or snack a couple of hours before bed. The more empty your stomach, the better. This can be difficult with how often you need to eat with my diet, but it is definitely possible. Find what works with your schedule.

Systemic Enzyme Dosages

This is a tough question because different companies have different amounts of enzymes in each pill. A standard dose is 5-10 pills, three times a day. Remember that you cannot overdose on these enzymes, so do not be afraid to up the dose. I have heard of people taking 20 pills, three times a day, when they are in extreme pain. Follow what it says on the bottle, and then increase the dose until you see desirable results.

Fish Oil

This one is required. If you are in pain, take fish oil. I like the Costco brand because it is cheap and works great. It is also from a good source. This stuff is as potent as NSAIDs in some studies, but without the horrible side effects (and it does not stop "good inflammation", which we still need).

How to take Fish Oil

The amount to take varies, but it is hard to take too much. Follow what it says on the bottle, and then increase the dosage slowly. I have heard of people comfortably taking as much as 9000mg a day, with absolutely no problems. Start small, and work your way up. Some say that they do not like taking fish oil because they have a couple "fish oil burps" after they take it. That is no excuse to not take one of the best pain relieving supplements on the market. Deal with the burps, and keep taking it.

MSM

There are books written about this mineral and how it helps chronic pain. I find this one to be an absolute requirement if you are in chronic pain. It is a type of sulpher that used to be present in our rain water years ago, but now it is not. That means it is not in our fruits and vegetables. Our diet lacks this mineral almost entirely. It is extremely safe and would be nearly impossible to overdose on it. One thing that this mineral helps with is edema. This is because its main function in the body is to make certain membranes more permeable. This means that nutrients and wastes can get in and out of your tissues a lot more easily (which means faster healing).

How to take MSM

Because of its low toxicity, you can take a lot of this supplement. It is not uncommon to take 1000mg, six times a day (Try to shoot for this dose). Small dosages throughout the day help with absorption. Buy MSM in bulk to save money. It is an extremely cheap supplement that you should take for as long as possible.

Magnesium

Calcium is needed by muscles to contract, and magnesium is needed by the muscles to relax. If you have tight muscles, chronic muscle, ligament, or tendon injuries, or bone issues, you need to start taking magnesium now. If not, you should take it anyways. This is another supplement that I feel should be required in your diet. Its uses are widespread in the body. Start taking it as soon as you are able.

How to take Magnesium

- Start taking at least 400mg a day.
- Drink with plenty of water.
- Sometimes it has the effects of a laxative if you take too much. This is common. If you get this effect, take a smaller dosage.

Try to get a magnesium supplement with multiple forms of magnesium. There are tons of different kinds of magnesium. The best ones are: Magnesium Glycinate, Citrate, Aspartate, Chloride, Lactate, Orotate, and Chelated forms. Any of these will do.

Vitamin D

Extremely important, and almost everyone in America today is deficient in this vitamin alone. It has a vast amount of functions in the human body, and if you are suffering from chronic pain, you are probably more deficient than the already deficient population of people around you. Some argue that vitamin D acts as a hormone in the body, and the fact that people are extremely deficient seems to correlate with the rise of many diseases and cancers that are common today. This is another vitamin that has so many purposes in the body that it is beyond the scope of this book to list them all. Some will start taking this vitamin and notice reduced pain in a week or so. This one is super safe to take, and extremely cheap. Give this one a shot and keep taking it if you feel better.

How to take Vitamin D

Be sure to buy Vitamin D3. Vitamin D2 is unsafe and more toxic. It is more possible to overdose on Vitamin D2. I find that taking 5000 I.U.s is the safest and most effective amount. Some people take 50,000 and other people take 500. It is up to you because there are no "perfect doses" found in the medical literature. Also, try to get vitamin D by soaking up some sunshine. The kind of vitamin D your body produces from the sun stays in the blood for twice as long as the kind that you ingest in supplement form. The best dosage for getting sunlight vitamin D is to show as much skin as possible, and lay out until you start to get pink. Be sure not to get sunburn!

Digestive Enzymes

These are required by the body to absorb every kind of vitamin, mineral, and basic nutrient out there. You need enzymes. Your body produces a lot of enzymes via the pancreas, but if you take enzymes with your food, it lightens the load on the pancreas. Remember, enzymes are hard to construct in the body, so if you take them in addition to a healthy diet, you are really giving your body a break so that it can focus its energy on the things that matter, such as chronic injuries.

How to take digestive enzymes

These enzymes, unlike systemic enzymes, do not need to be enterically coated.

Take 1-2 digestive enzyme pills at every meal.

Turmeric

Turmeric is the most effective and well known herb for inflammation. I find the best way to ingest it is to buy the root, then juice it. You can take it in pill form, or powder, but it does not have nearly as much "kick" as when it is in raw form. This is another one of those supplements that helps your body fight inflammation in a million ways. It is best just to throw this on your shopping list for now until forever. It has a pungent taste, but you will get used to it fast. There is no ideal dosage. Just eat as much turmeric as you can.

Protease Enzymes

These are the systemic enzymes, but in isolated forms. For example, most systemic enzymes have all of these enzymes and more in combination. But when you walk into the vitamin store, you may not be able to find systemic enzymes if they do not have that great of a selection (but they are extremely easy to find online). If you want to try out enzyme therapy, then you can try one of the enzymes listed below to see how they work for you. These isolated enzymes are usually pretty cheap, and will give you favorable results. Proteases are famous for reducing swelling, reducing pain, and speeding up healing times. The results will not be as good as a fully-fledged systemic enzymes, but they do help. Some common protease enzymes available in the stores are:

- Bromelain
- Papain
- Trypsin/Chymotrypsin
- Pancreatin

I have found that Bromelain is the most common and well-studied protease available on the market. All of them will give you favorable results if you are in pain regardless. One difference that you will find is that most systemic enzymes are enterically coated. This is a good thing to have, and some protease enzyme supplements have this, but not all. Try to choose the one that says "enterically coated" on the front of the bottle or box.

How to take Protease enzyme supplements

- They have to be taken on an empty stomach. Try to take them an hour before a meal.
- Try to buy enterically coated protease enzyme supplements.
- Take 5-10 tablets three times a day.

Glucosamine/Chondroitin

This supplement is well studied and extremely safe. This one is crucial for pain induced by cartilage damage. Even though glucosamine and chondroitin are separate supplements, they are almost always sold together. This supplement helps inflammation in various ways as well and speeds up healing.

How to take Glucosamine/Chondroitin

It is an extremely safe supplement with no adverse side effects reported in the medical literature. I would start with whatever the bottle says, and increase the dose gradually to around double that of what is stated on the bottle. There are studies that mention taking 1/3 a pound of pure glucosamine every day for over a year without adverse reactions. That would be like taking multiple bottles every single day. Doubling your dose is completely safe and will give you good results. I like the Costco brand because it guarantees potency and is much cheaper than the competitors.

First Step of MSTR:

Release the Trigger Points

Trigger points are tender spots of tissue in the muscle that are made in response to any and all structural injuries in the body. Their purpose is to cause pain when you move a damaged area of the body. This is to force you to rest so that your body can fix the damage in the injury. These trigger points are great for fixing normal injures and forcing someone to rest, but if you have a chronic injury (anything over six weeks), the trigger points are causing you more harm than good.

The best way to find these trigger points is to carefully feel around the areas I suggest for each injury and try to find tender areas that hurt to rub. What we want to do is slowly rub each trigger point with blunt force until it is less tender. When it is less tender, or the muscle itself feels more soft, then we know we are done. For some muscles this can be a slow but forceful rub with 6 to 12 slow strokes (a slow and focused massage).

Sometimes rubbing a trigger point will have a "good pain", like when you get knots massaged out of your back. The key to releasing trigger points is to not apply too much pressure. It is best not to go more than 6 out of 10 on the pain scale, where 0 is no pain, and 10 is the most pain.

When we are in chronic pain, and find that trigger point therapy can reduce our pain, some of us will rub the trigger points too hard in a desperate attempt to get rid of the pain. It is much better to keep at 6 out of 10 on the pain scale, and do a lot of consistent small sessions of trigger point work, than it is to do an inconsistent number of "hard" sessions. 3 small sessions a day is much better for you than 1 hard session once a day.

Using tools will allow you to use more pressure on a trigger point than you can with just your hands. I also suggest trying to use tools whenever you can in order to avoid using your thumbs. Thumbs can be damaged from using them too much to rub out trigger points. The last thing we need is more injuries when we have a chronic injury!

The pictures in this chapter will show guidelines of where common trigger points will be for individual muscles. Notice that the pictures included in this book do not show pain referral patterns. This is because we are not going to be chasing the pain referrals. A trigger point pain referral is pain caused by a trigger point, but far away from the actual trigger point. Your job is to use the pictures in this chapter to find the individual trigger points causing your pain, and rub them out until they are not as tender. If you need to know which muscles you need to treat, check out the chapter on "individual injuries" to figure out what muscles are causing your pain.

Some people will have to hit all the trigger points I suggest for an injury; some will only have a couple of active trigger points. Sometimes you will not only find a tender spot, but you might find a small nodule or lump or tight band in the muscle as well. This is what a trigger point feels like. You need to slowly massage this out until it is not as tender as when you started. Rubbing them back and forth is the best way to do this. Rub them nice and slowly. If you apply too much pressure to these little trigger points, you will have more pain and more problems. If you massage them nice and softly and have a medium amount of pain while doing so, you will have less pain and fewer problems with your injury. If you do not feel a tender spot, try pushing harder and deeper into the tissues. Sometimes they like to hide pretty deep inside a muscle.

Remember, trigger points will be there NO MATTER WHAT. If you have chronic pain from inflammation or injury, there is a trigger point that is nearby and active to the injury that is causing more pain. If you do not get pain relief with trigger point therapy, you are either not looking in the right area, or you are not pushing hard enough. Keep looking around and push deeper!

One extra thing to know about trigger points is that they cause "referred pain patterns". This means that when you have active trigger points in one part of your body, it will automatically send pain signals to another part of the body, even if the injury is already healed! This is why I suggest doing trigger point therapies first and foremost to see what kind of results you get. For some, these trigger point methods will practically "fix" you. For most, they need to be done consistently until your chronic pain is gone.

If you have fibromyalgia or myofascial pain syndrome, you should probably find a trigger point pain referral guide so that you can figure out which muscles are causing your pain, and chase after those.

In this book, I show exactly which muscles are most likely dysfunctional for your given injury by following the "individual injury" chapter later on in this book. Each injury area will have a list of muscles that you need to treat daily. Some of the muscles, or possibly even all of the muscles, will more than likely have trigger points.

My favorite way to finding the hard-to-find trigger points is by feeling the other side of your body. If your right forearm more than likely has trigger points from your injury, but your left forearm is healthy, feel the left forearm to see how a "healthy" muscle should feel like. You will quickly find that a healthy muscle is soft and malleable. A dysfunctional muscle will be more stiff and hard and will have little lumps, knots, or taught bands hiding inside the muscle. Those are the trigger points.

After a few sessions of trigger point therapy, you may feel like your tender spots have become less sensitive and that you might be fine without any more trigger point work. This is wrong. Keep feeling around the muscles and search for new trigger points. Sometimes after doing the superficial (surface) layer of muscles, you will later find a whole new set of trigger points deeper in the muscle. These ones will usually require more focused pressure in order to release them. If you are not seeing results, try pushing a bit harder. Just keep with it daily and do not give up!

You can do these trigger point release methods any time throughout the day. If you are in a lot of pain, doing them 6 times a day is fine (6 light sessions is better than 1 intense session a day). If the area becomes extremely sore or feels more tender, let the area rest and come back to it in a day or two. Your body will adapt to the trigger point therapy quickly, and it is not unusual for you to be able to double the amount of therapy sessions and pressure that you use on the trigger points in as little as 2-3 weeks. It is important to slowly ease into the treatments and to build up to more sessions and more applied pressure while massaging. Listen to your body and respond accordingly.

Trigger Point Tools

It is great to use your hands for diagnostic evaluation of a muscle in question and we will use our hands to deactivate the trigger points, but it is much more ideal to use a trigger point tool when you can. A tool will do quite a few things at once:

- Focus the mechanical pressure to a small area, thus going deeper and also getting hard-to-find trigger points.

- Save our hands from damage. Pressing into trigger points six times a day can beat your hands up pretty quickly and cause more issues. Avoid this at all costs!

- Some tools work well for some muscles, and not so well for others. Use the muscle guides ahead to understand which tools are best suited for releasing certain trigger points.

The following pages contain common trigger point tools that we will use in this book. Most of them are available online and at economical prices.

Lacrosse Ball

This is my favorite trigger point therapy tool. It is small, light, and effective and can be used on nearly all muscles if you get creative. I love pushing my body weight against the ball when it is placed against a wall or on the ground. It is extremely useful and nearly required for work in the gluteal region. I cannot recommend this tool more. It is crazy cheap and lasts forever. By the way, do not use a tennis ball; they are HORRIBLE for trigger point massage.

Rolling Pin

This is extremely useful for getting rid of dysfunction in calf and quadriceps musculature. It is nearly required for knee pain trigger point sessions throughout the day. The number one thing you MUST get when buying a rolling pin for trigger point therapy is one that has ball bearings. If it does not, you will be disappointed and frustrated with your results. There are lots of "roller massage" sticks on the market, but a 10 dollar rolling pin works just as well as those high-priced massage sticks.

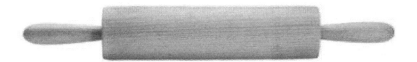

The Back Buddy ©

This tool is nearly required for all kinds of back, hip, and neck pain. It is one of my favorite tools. It is really useful for self therapy if you do not have someone around (especially when you must do 6 small trigger point sessions a day). I also find it better than a trigger point therapist in some ways because you can find exact trigger point locations and be able to rub them out accordingly.

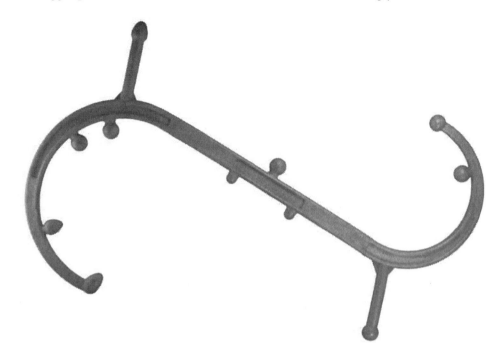

<u>Pros:</u>

- Sturdy, does not flex like other massage sticks even if you are using it to massage really deep.

- Great for places you cannot reach. I can reach gluteal muscles and hard to reach back muscles. I can also use the various little knobs to massage Infraspinatus and Subscapularis.

- Great assortment of different knobs in very well thought-out places. One side has rounded knobs for a light massage, and the other end has pointy knobs so you can go REALLY deep into the tissues.

- Because it is an "S" design, you can use one end to massage your back, glutes, and neck and then hook the other end of the "S" to a pole, stick or something stationary so you can lean back and put your weight into the massage. This is great for deep gluteal muscles that need a lot of pressure to reach.

<u>Cons:</u>

- It is heavy. If your arms are extremely weak from a shoulder injury, it may be hard to use at first.

- Hard to bring with you everywhere you go. I leave mine on the side of my seat in my car so I can always get to it easily.

- Hard to get used to for some. It can take some practice to be able to use it. There are so many ways to use this stick that it is hard to find the ways that best help you at first.

Tip: If you need to massage your back, and you are in your car, put one end of the stick around your back, and the other end of the stick around the steering wheel. This makes it so you can lean your whole weight into the massage stick. I do not suggest using this on small muscles or neck muscles.

The Knobble©

This tool is great to use in areas where you would commonly use your hands. It is an even better tool if you can get someone to use one on your trigger points. The only downside is that you must exert muscular force to push the tool into your body (unless someone is doing it to you).

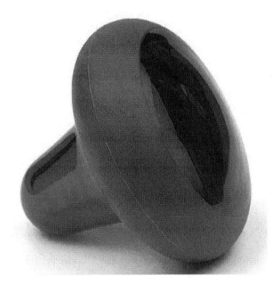

Foam Roller

This tool is nearly required for all hip and knee issues. It is great for releasing quadriceps musculature (especially Vastus Lateralis!) and many others. It is very important to get a large diameter foam roller and a small diameter "travel size" foam roller so you can hit different muscles with different amounts of pressure.

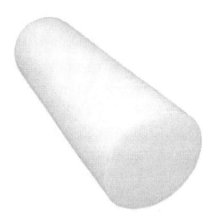

Wooden Foot Roller

These are nearly required for all foot and ankle issues; it's also good for some knee issues. They release all the muscles on the bottom of the foot, better than any other tool out there. I highly recommend it.

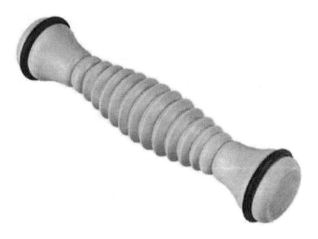

Air Hockey Apparatus

These things are great for back muscles and so much more. You can use it in place of a Knobble©.

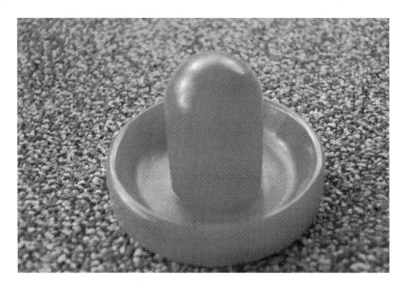

My favorite homemade tool:

Find some sort of rounded peg. Then find a small piece of wood. Drill hole in wood and put peg into hole with glue. Now you have one of the best massage tools on the planet! You can use this for all sorts of trigger points on the body. It is great for using as a back erector trigger point massager.

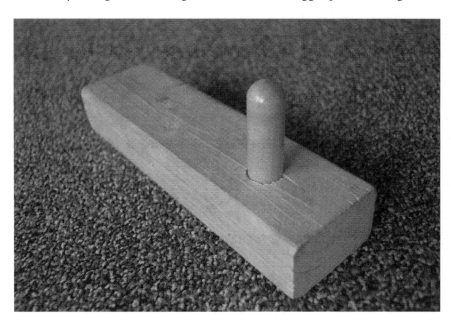

Second Step of MSTR:

Release the Fascia Adhesions

This one is a bit tricky, but once you master this technique, it will set you up for a LOT of relief from your pain. This method also makes the results you see from your trigger point releasing more "permanent" and gives the trigger points less of a reason to come back.

Why release the fascia?

The trigger points we released earlier are bundles of muscle fibers that are held tight in a chronically contracted state. Around these muscle fibers, there is connective tissue (fascia) that structurally holds the muscle fibers together. When the trigger points are locked in place for a long time, the fascia tightens around the trigger points until the fascia is tight as well. The fascia needs to be released if you want your trigger point therapy results to stay. Once you release the trigger points, it is MUCH easier to release the fascia. The way we do this is by scraping the tissues with a plastic or metal edge. What you want is something that can apply very direct pressure to a tissue, but not damage the skin. Rounded edges work best.

Scraping guidelines:

The muscles, tendons, and ligaments need to be relaxed and/or stretched in order to release the fascia around them. This is done by contracting the opposite side of the body part you are working with. When you release the calf muscle fascia, you need to make sure your shin muscle is contracted. To do this, bring the top of your foot as high up as you can toward the shin. This will stretch the calf muscle and make it easier to scrape.

Another example of this is when you release the bottom of the foot's fascia, you need to pull your toes back as far as you can with one hand, and then scrape the bottom of the foot with the other hand. Follow these guidelines for every area of the body.

Also experiment. Surprisingly, some muscles prefer different amounts of stretch to release them. Most of them prefer to be completely stretched, others like it better when the muscle is only partially stretched. Try stretching the muscle different amounts while scraping to see what works best for you.

Some injuries do not require too much scraping. Others will require a lot of scraping. It all depends on what I recommend at the end of the book in the "Individual Injuries" section. Use this section to figure out which muscles you need to scrape.

USE LUBRICATION. Any lotion will work usually. Put it all over the area being treated. DO NOT SCRAPE WITHOUT! You need the lubrication so that you do not damage the skin and so that the tool works properly to break up the adhesions.

The pictures ahead will show where a muscle is. This is where you will do light passes over first. You want to hit the whole muscle and check to see if there is any dysfunctional fascia in the full length of the muscle. Next, check out the muscles pictures ahead for circle areas. These circle areas are likely places to find dysfunctional fascia. Usually these areas will have quite a lot of adhesions, and it will be your job to scrape them out.

If a muscle has excessive amounts of trigger points where the whole muscle is contracted and stiff, it is wise to just stick with trigger point therapy for now and work on scraping later.

When you first scrape a full muscle, you will use equal pressure over the whole muscle, and scrape the whole thing. The end goal is to do a few passes with moderate pressure. After the whole muscle is warmed up, you can go over the circle areas which will more than likely have an abundance of scar tissue that needs to be dealt with.

Remember that most people will have scar tissue in different places. It is your goal to find the areas of dysfunction for your given injury, and deal with them accordingly.

Not all muscles can be scraped. The muscle guide will tell you if the muscle should be scraped or not.

First, you will want to start scraping with a few light pressure passes and slowly build up to moderate pressure. After a few sessions of scraping, you can build up to more extreme amounts of pressure. Try to go a little harder each time. This does not mean hurt yourself! Do what is comfortable, but be a bit aggressive with the pressure. Even if it feels really good to scrape, do not scrape more than 10-20 times per area. The best rule of thumb is to stop when the area is less tender.

Do these every day after one of your trigger point therapy sessions, but not as often as the trigger point therapies. Even if you are doing 6 sessions of trigger point therapy, do only 1 session of scraping. Once your body adapts to this therapy, you will be able to increase the amount of sessions and the amount of pressure applied. If anything feels more tender or sore, take a day or two of rest, and ease back into it.

You will probably hear noises when you scrape the muscles. This is good! It means that you are finding adhesions in the tissue and are releasing them.

The texture that you will look for in the tissues is a "grainy" texture. If you were to scrape over a healthy area, it would feel nice and smooth. When you scrape a structure that has dysfunctional fascia, it will feel rough and grainy from all the adhesions. These areas are where you want to focus your pressure. Try to rub out the grains by passing the tools more over these areas.

A great way to find "grainy" areas with scar tissue is to lightly scrape the area in question. If it is nice and smooth, then it is more than likely functional and healthy. This does not mean that it does not have trigger points! This only applies to finding cross-link adhesions in the fascia. If you hear a bunch of noises and you feel lots of tiny bumps when you run your scraping tools over the area, than you know you hit some dysfunctional fascia that has to be taken care of.

It is important to go slowly and not force anything. It can be a little painful at times to do this therapy, especially if your injury has been around for a long time, but it just means you must ease very carefully into the scraping methods. Do not think that more pressure is better. After you find the dysfunctional areas, scraping really hard in a desperate attempt to fix yourself will not work. The changes that scraping invokes will take days to weeks of consistent work before you will notice amazing results. Start your scraping methods off soft and keep building up pressure slowly.

Scraping Tools: How to Pick the Right Tools for Breaking up Adhesions in the Fascia

There are different areas of the body that respond to different kinds of scraping angles, pressures, tools, and etc. You can buy these tools online, but most are extremely expensive - literally hundreds to thousands of dollars for things you can easily replace with household objects. The expensive ones bought by doctors have got to be the biggest scam in the medical world today and it drives me crazy. You can buy cheaper versions of these tools online and they go by the name of "gua sha" tools, but I am almost sure that you can find a better makeshift tool in your kitchen right now.

One thing that all the tools used for this therapy have in common is the edge. You want a rounded edge to safely scrape an area. It should be plastic or metal. Plastic rounded edges are easier to find. Metal ones are better, but harder to find in household objects.

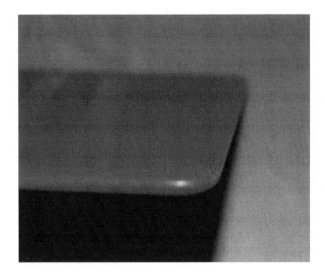

Some areas of the body are small, like the forearm, and require small tools. Other areas of the body that are larger, such as the thigh, respond a lot better with bigger tools. Some areas respond better with curved tools, such as concave and convex curves. Concave angles are great for sensitive areas, or areas that fit the concave curve. Convex curved tools work better for getting in extra deep and for breaking up a localized area of scar tissue (a muscle origin or attachment, for example).

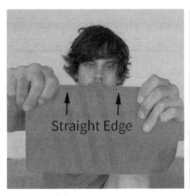

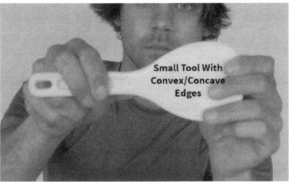

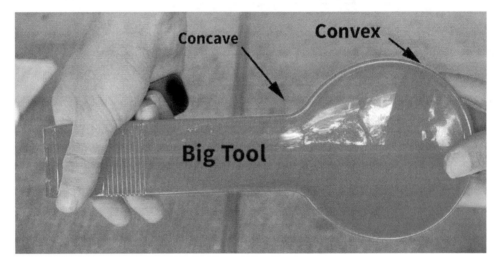

The Muscle Guide

Now you know how to deal with trigger points and dysfunctional fascia (in a theoretical sense). This muscle guide is your personal guide to finding these dysfunctional areas. You will use the guide to find out where these trigger points and dysfunctional fascia are located. All of the muscles are in alphabetical order.

IMPORTANT-

What you must do now is go to the chapter on **"Individual Injuries"** and figure out which muscles you need to work on. Then, come back to this muscle guide and look at only the muscles I mention for each injury. There are a lot of muscles in this section, but if you have only one injury, you only have to work on a few muscles. After you find out which muscles you need to work on, bookmark the pages describing their treatment. You will need to come back to these bookmarks daily.

The next few pages have information on the directional terms that you need to understand in navigating through the muscle guides descriptions.

Note: You do not need to memorize the huge names of the muscles!! You just need to know what their name is so you can come back to this muscle guide and find them. Do not be intimidated by the size of these words, and you do not need to know much about them except for where they are located and where the trigger points/scraping areas are.

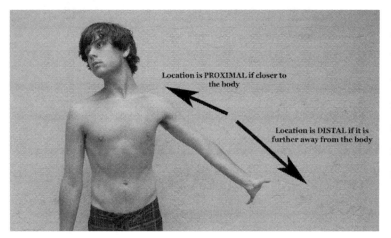

One thing to understand in "navigating" through this chapter is that some of the words will be a little foreign to you. The most important set of directional terms you need to familiarize yourself with is "proximal" and "distal".

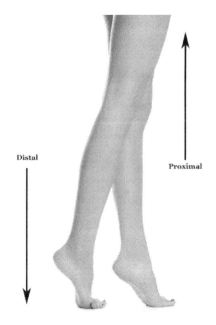

- Proximal is closer to the "core" of the body (closer to the spine).

- Distal is further from the core of the body, and references things as closer to the toes and fingers.

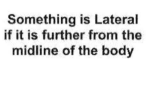
Something is Lateral
if it is further from the
midline of the body

Another directional term you should familiarize yourself with is medial/lateral. Medial is toward the midline of the body, and lateral is outward and away from the body.

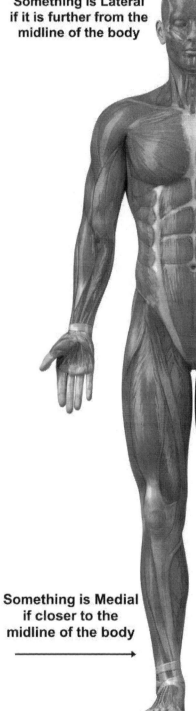
Something is Medial
if closer to the
midline of the body

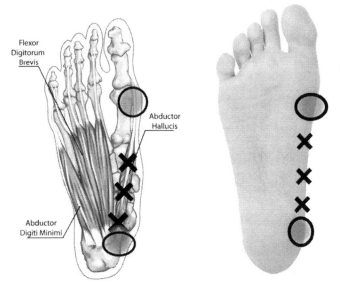

Abductor Hallucis

This muscle is nearly required to work on if you have plantar fasciitis or other foot and ankle issues. The reason why is because there is a nerve and set of blood vessels that tuck right under the muscle. If these blood vessels and/or nerves become entrapped because of dysfunction in this muscle, then areas of the foot will become numb / weak and/or their blood supply will become hindered (causing stagnation and much more). This muscle is extremely important for proper walking gait mechanics. If it is dysfunctional for a long time, it can cause issues elsewhere.

Trigger Point Treatment:
The best way to treat this muscles trigger points is with a foot roller or lacrosse ball (foot roller more ideal). Just softly roll your foot back and forth on the inner edge of your foot.

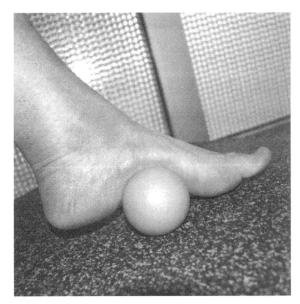

Scraping Treatment:

I like to use a big tool with a concave curve to fit around the curvature of the muscle. Be sure to deal with the mass of scar tissue that loves to develop at both attachment points. One is right behind the big toe, and the other is right at the front of the heel bone (Calcaneus).

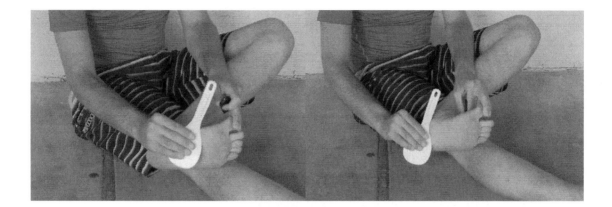

Adductor Brevis/Longus

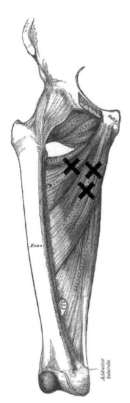

These muscles can be very sensitive when you first work on them, but they respond well to MSTR. There are lots of nerves in the area, and if you want to scrape, you need to be careful. Feel the tissue with your hands and try light scraping if you think it is warranted. If it is grainy, then go in deeper, but not very deep. It is better

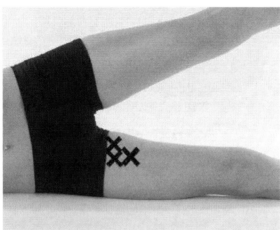

to do distal to proximal (from knee to hip) scraping motions because of all the lymph vessels in the area. I prefer sticking to just trigger point therapy for both of these muscles.

Trigger Point Treatment:
A big foam roller works best. Go on your hands and knees, lift one leg up and stick the foam roller under it. Your legs will be in a "frog leg" position. Try to roll all the way up the leg to the attachment point on the pelvis and down the length of both muscles. There are some nerves nearby and they cause a different feeling. Trigger point pain has a distinct feeling. If you feel a "scary" kind of pain, it is probably a nerve and you need to reduce the pressure.

Scraping Treatment:
Depends. Sometimes it is needed, but for most situations I would just stick with trigger point therapy. Try soft and light strokes to see what the texture of the tissue is like. You will not be able to really scrape the muscles, but it is possible to break up some superficial adhesions in the fascia around the muscle (which loves to adhere to nearby structures). Use a large tool with a concave or straight edge.

Adductor Magnus

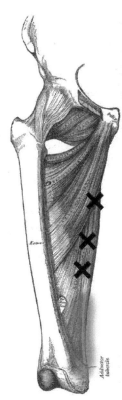

This one is similar to the other adductor muscles and needs a big foam roller to do trigger point work on. The only difference is that this muscle goes from the pelvis and extends all the way down to the knee (right above the knee, attaches to adductor tubercle). If you are working on the gracilis, you will be working on this

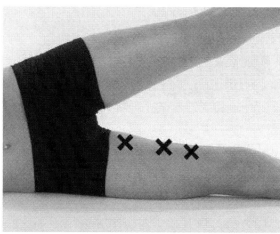

muscle. It is very long like the gracilis and will be pretty sensitive at first.

Trigger Point Treatment:

Responds well to trigger point therapy and usually is taken care of in about a week of consistent trigger point sessions. I would do this muscle at most 2-3 times a day and ease into it at first. After it is more functional, it likes to stay that way for awhile unless you have a pretty severe injury. Use a foam roller, a nice big one, and roll out the length of the muscle.

Scraping Treatment:

As with all adductors, be very gentle. Less nerves at the distal portions of this muscle makes it easier to scrape than adductor longus/brevis. Just be sure to go slowly at first and build up pressure. The adductor tubercle is notorious for having dysfunctional fascia (see big circle area in picture). As with the trigger points, the fascia responds well and likes to stay that way as long as perpetuating factors are taken care of. Use a big tool with a concave or straight edge.

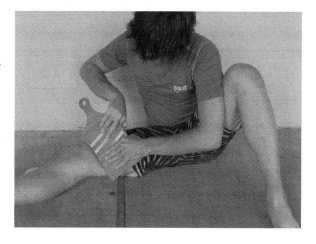

Back Erectors

These are dysfunctional in people that have back pain. This does not mean they are to blame for your back pain, even though they are your back muscles. They are one muscle of many that need to be treated. The back muscles are very important to treat, just as important as all the other muscles that stabilize the spine. If you have chronic back pain, the fascia in this area will be extremely dysfunctional. This is a common area for having issues, so follow all the advice ahead to make these muscles work more properly.

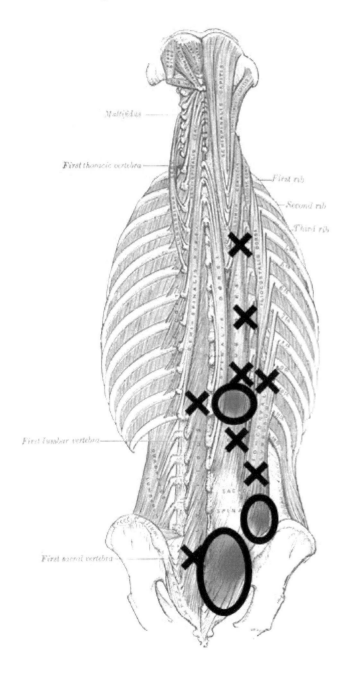

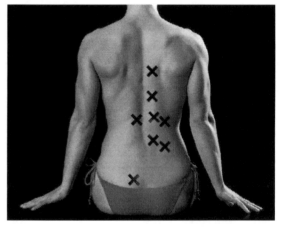

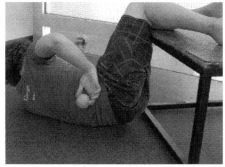

Trigger Point Treatment:
One or two lacrosse balls are the best for fixing these areas trigger points. Put them on the ground and roll your back over them slowly. It is even better to put your feet up on a small box or chair so that the muscles relax even further. Do not use a foam roller over the lower back, only for the upper and mid back areas.

Another great way to get the trigger points to release is with The Back Buddy © stick. This stick gets right in the areas you want and you can use the stick as a lever to push a lot of mechanical pressure into the area.

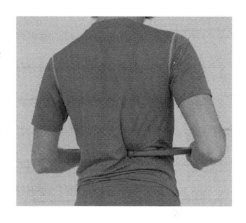

Another tool I love to release this muscle with is by using an electric shiatsu massage chair. These tools, unlike our hands, never get tired. For an added effect, lay the massage chair on the ground so that you have to lay your whole weight into the chair, then let the massage chair work out any trigger points it finds.

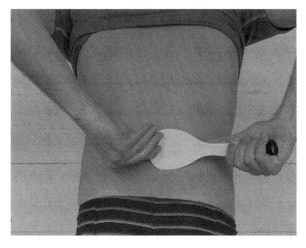

Scraping Treatment:
The whole area responds nicely. The spots right above the pelvis bone and sacrum are very important because this area is filled with dense fascia that attaches many different muscles together. These thick fascia areas love to become really dense and filled with adhesions if you have chronic back pain. I suggest scraping only when the area is relaxed rather than stretched. In chronic lower back pain, the area will become so filled with adhesions that the skin will be tacked down to the underlying layers of fascia, causing further dysfunction. If you pull the skin on a healthy athlete's back, it will be able to do so easily and will be soft and supple. If you do this "skin pinch test" to someone with lower back pain, it will be tough to lift up and will be denser. After a couple sessions of scraping, this will go away and you should be able to pull the skin up with less effort. The whole back also responds well to cupping therapies (an old Chinese therapy where cups are attached to the back with suction). This therapy pulls the skin up so that the tight fascia will release to a degree and become more functional.

Biceps Brachii

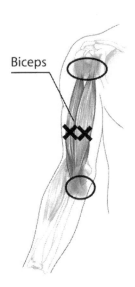

Biceps

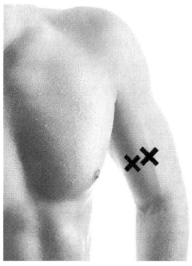

It is really common for this muscle to become dysfunctional and cause elbow and shoulder pain. It is overworked in lots of athletes which leads to muscle imbalances. The long head of this muscle travels in a small sheath near the shoulder and attaches to the scapula. This area is prone to injury and ruptures are not uncommon. The distal portion attaches to an aponeurosis (tendon sheath) that covers the forearm flexors. The problem with that structure (biceptual aponeurosis) is that it lies extremely close to the median nerve. When it becomes entrapped in this area, symptoms of carpal tunnel syndrome can appear. This muscle is also commonly dysfunctional in office workers.

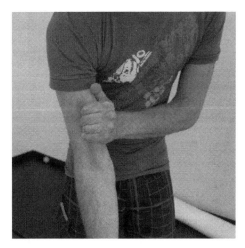

Trigger Point Treatment:

Every area of this muscle is easy to palpate, so trigger point therapy is pretty easily done. You can usually use your hands for the treatments if you do not use your thumbs (grab the muscle with the fingers). It is easy to find tender points in this muscle and they can respond pretty quickly to treatment. If you have long-standing tendonosis (of either insertion), it can take the muscle a few weeks to become completely functional again.

Scraping Treatment:

Scrape the attachment points of the muscle. Using a small convex shaped tool, scrape the tendons of attachment and the biceptual aponeurosis. These areas are extremely common spots for dysfunctional fascia. Use a small convex tool for the superior attachment to the shoulder.

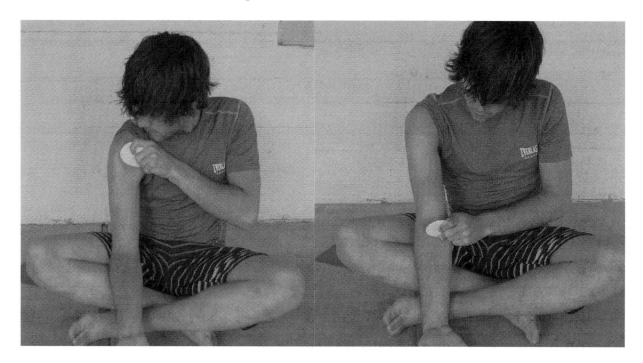

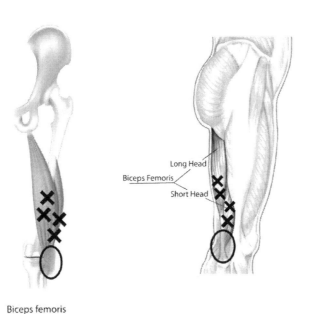 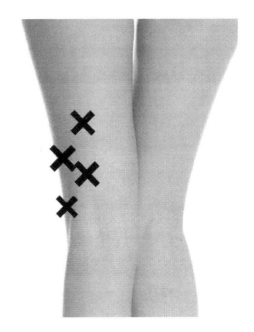

Biceps femoris

Biceps Femoris

This muscle controls the rotation and flexion of the knee and must be treated if long standing knee issues have been present. If you have a sedentary job or lifestyle, this muscle becomes shortened and causes problems in lower back, pelvis, knee, and foot biomechanics.

Trigger Point Treatment:

Small foam roller works well under the thigh while seated or two lacrosse balls under the thigh while being seated on a flat bench or table. It is important to get the most outer portion of the muscle which controls knee rotation. This portion is easily accessible if you externally rotate your thigh. It's best to do this while seated, by lifting your foot inward towards the body's midline, or other leg, and rolling the outside hamstring portion (short head of Biceps Femoris) against a foam roller or lacrosse ball. Extremely important in knee pain patients!

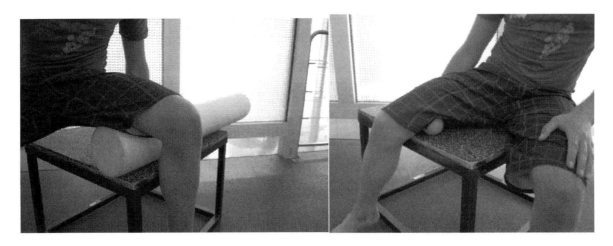

Scraping Treatment:

It is very helpful to scrape this muscle, especially at the distal portion (near the knee). This area loves to develop adhesions because of its huge demand to stabilize the knee joint. It is an easy area to scrape when someone else does it for you, but it is better to learn how to scrape it yourself. Knee must be extended in order to scrape this muscle.

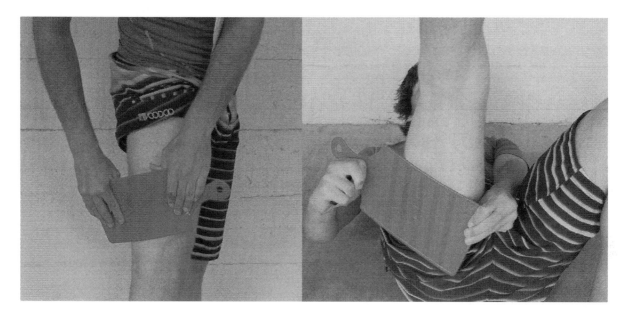

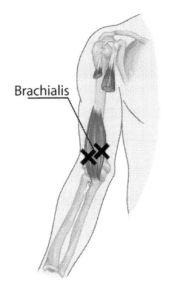

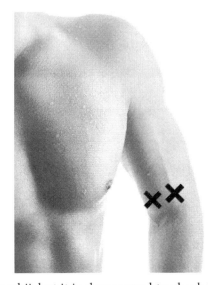

Brachialis

This muscle lies just under the Biceps Brachii muscle. This muscle only moves the elbow joint, and does not move or stabilize the shoulder joint how the Biceps Brachii does. This muscle is a primary mover of elbow flexion when the wrist is pronated. This muscle is not as commonly dysfunctional as the Biceps Brachii, but it is always good to check the condition of this muscle. The reason is because the Radial nerve passes through this muscle. If the muscle is dysfunctional, it can cause compression on the radial nerve. Usually trigger point therapy can fix this problem pretty easily. If you're having pain when you straighten your elbow, or pain in your thumb, give this muscle a second check for trigger points.

Trigger Point Treatment:
Lift up the Biceps Brachii muscle out of the way a little and you will feel most areas of the muscle. Watch out for nerves on the inside of the arm and radial nerve on the outside. If you stay right under the biceps Brachii, you will be good to go.

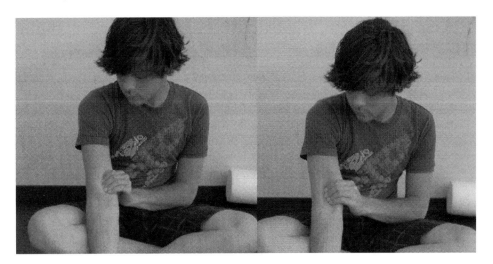

Scraping Treatment:

Not recommended. Stick to scraping the bicep brachii if area is severely dysfunctional. Too many nearby structures are too sensitive to warrant scraping. This muscle is very localized to the elbow, and dysfunction in the fascia is not as common as other muscles. But muscular problems in this muscle are very common.

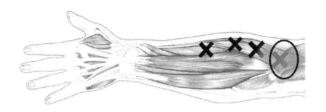

Brachioradialis/ Extensor Carpi Radialis Group/ Supinator

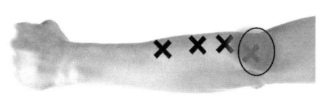

This is a big muscle bundle of the forearm that controls elbow joint and forearm rotation and wrist extension. If you have any kind of hand pain/wrist/elbow issues, it is good to check this area out. You will almost always find a trigger point in the proximal area of these muscles attachment. The trigger points of this muscle though are hard to differentiate from each other, so it is best to treat them as one area.

Trigger Point Treatment:
I think the best way to treat this is with the corner of a door. This works out all dysfunction in the muscle. If this is too much pressure, try using a lacrosse ball against a wall and lean your forearm into this area.

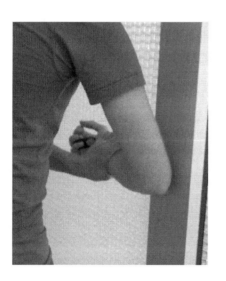

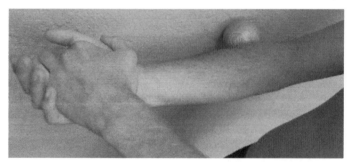

Scraping Treatment:

You really need to scrape the attachment point of this area if you find dysfunction in the muscles. This area is notorious for laying down adhesions and causing dysfunction. It is usually the weaker muscle group in muscle imbalances when it comes to the forearm and over time it adapts by laying down lots of scar tissue (cross-link adhesions). The best way to make sure you are getting the attachment point is to feel for the bony landmarks and find exactly where these muscles attach to bone, and scrape right there.

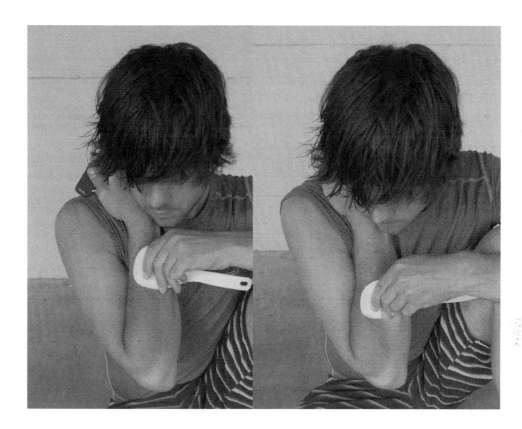

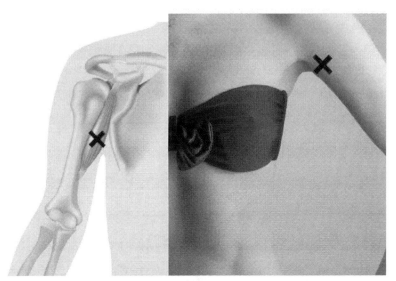

Coracobrachialis

This is a very important muscle to treat if you suffer from shoulder pain. This little muscle loves to cause a ton of pain when dysfunctional. It is responsible for raising your arm in front of you (flexion) and also assists in adduction of the shoulder joint. This muscle is hard to find. It lies under the deltoid and is medial (towards the midline of the body) to the biceps brachii.

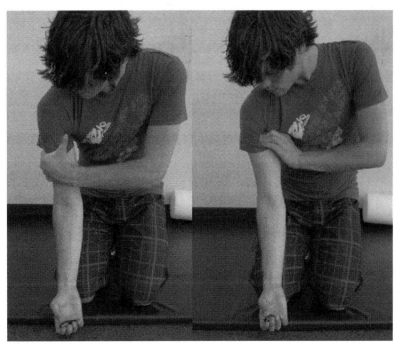

Trigger Point Treatment:
It is hard to find. It is a small muscle and does not require much force to release, so you can safely use your thumb without any problems. The muscle responds well to up and down and side-to-side massage very well. The only issue you may run into is hitting the nerve. There is a nerve that runs just posterior (towards your back) to the coracobrachialis. It will feel very sensitive if you hit it. Just make sure you progress to higher amounts of pressure slowly. You should be looking for a "tender point" that feels good to massage. If you hit an area that is tender but does not feel like the usual "feel good muscle massage" feeling, than you are on a nerve. Take a good look at the photo above to figure out the location of this muscle.

Scraping Treatment:
Because it is so close to a nerve, and because it is very deep, it is not smart to scrape this muscle. You can get great results by sticking to the trigger point therapy above.

Deltoid Muscle

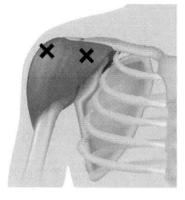 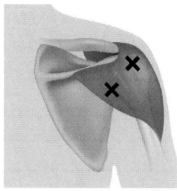

Anterior view   Posterior view

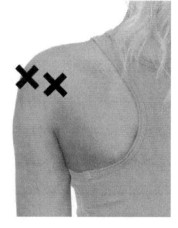 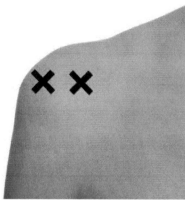

Deltoid

This is a very multi articulate muscle with a wide variety of movements. Muscle fiber in the deltoid start and end in various areas, and the muscle is extremely important for shoulder stability. Because the shoulder is very prone to instability issues, this muscle needs to be functioning properly to stabilize the shoulder joint.

Usually this muscle is not dysfunctional on its own, and dysfunction in this muscle is more of a side effect of having dysfunction in other muscles, such as the Pectoralis Major, Scalene muscles, and Rotator Cuff muscles.

Trigger Point Treatment:
The best way to treat all the trigger points of this muscle is without a doubt by using a lacrosse ball against a wall.

Scraping Treatment:
This muscle is fixed pretty easily from trigger point therapy so you usually do not have to scrape it. I think it is good to scrape the muscle if you had a surgery months ago when you have scars because they had to cut through the deltoid. This scraping will help out all the post-surgery induced dysfunction in this muscle greatly.

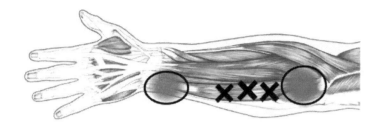

Extensor Carpi Ulnaris

If you have wrist pain, you should check this muscle out. It is a strong muscle and is overworked from typing, but it is easily treated.

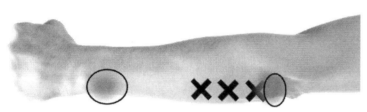

Trigger Point Treatment:
Use the corner of a door to rub out all the dysfunctional trigger points out of this muscle. If you want a slightly less aggressive massage, use a lacrosse ball against a wall and push your forearm and bodyweight against the ball in the area of the muscle.

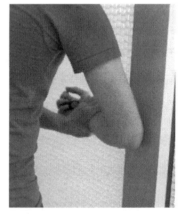

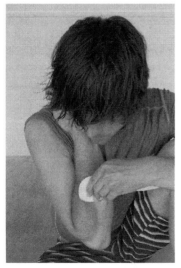

Scraping Treatment:
Ulnar nerves passes near this muscle, so not smart to do aggressive scraping. I find that it is useful to do soft passes over this muscle though and works well to break up any small adhesions that have developed. When scraping this muscle, just go soft and scrape the whole muscle a couple times.

Extensor Digitorum

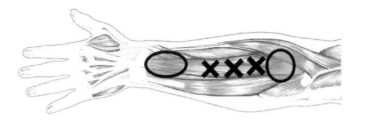

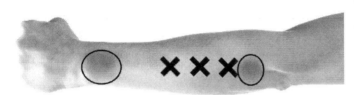

This is an important muscle that commonly has dysfunctional tissue. It responds quickly to treatment. It is usually weak compared to the flexor side of the forearm and if the muscular balance is too extreme, then the wrist is not as stable as it should be, causing long-term issues.

Trigger Point Treatment:
Use the corner of a door to rub out all the dysfunctional trigger points out of this muscle. If you want a slightly less aggressive massage, use a lacrosse ball against a wall and push your forearm and bodyweight against the ball in the area of the muscle.

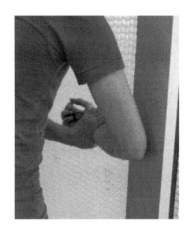

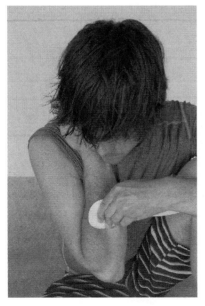

Scraping Treatment:
Go over the whole muscle. The belly of this muscle seems to have some adhesions and responds well to scraping.

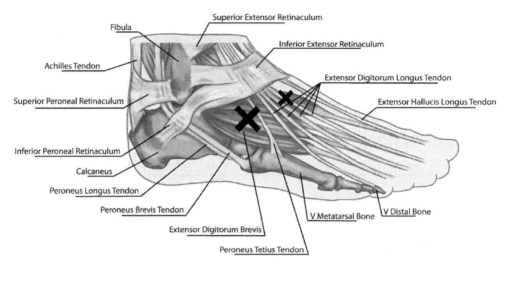

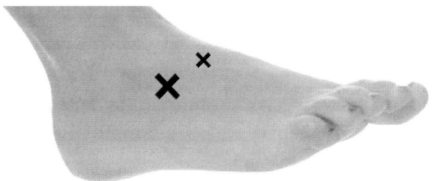

Extensor Hallucis/Digitorum Group

This is a very small muscle group on the top of the foot. It can become dysfunctional if your walking gait has been bad for a long time due to an injury or other causes. You can find these muscles by looking for a soft spot of muscle on top of the foot.

Trigger Point Treatment:
This muscle is very easy to treat. It is extremely small and responds well to just rubbing them out with your hand. It does not take that much pressure to get rid of the trigger points in these muscles.

Scraping Treatment:
Not needed due to nerves nearby and lack of fascia dysfunction in this area.

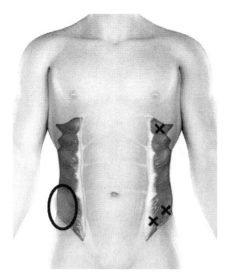

Abdominal Group (External and Internal Abdominal Oblique)

This is a key muscle group of the "spiral line" kinetic chain and when dysfunctional can literally twist the body and keep it there.

This muscle group is responsible for proper breathing function and needs to be working properly. Luckily, it is not commonly dysfunctional. It is usually more weak than dysfunctional, and some people will benefit greatly from doing some abdominal workouts, especially if they have back pain that originates from excessive anterior pelvic tilt.

Trigger Point Treatment:

This location is home to a handful of randomly-placed trigger points. Just feel around the area while your hands are on your stomach and feel for the typical tender spots. You should be lying down while doing this, and breathing slowly and with full breaths. Be sure to relax.

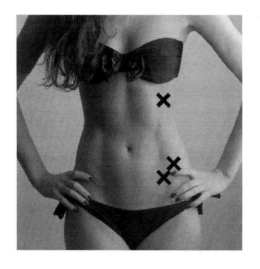

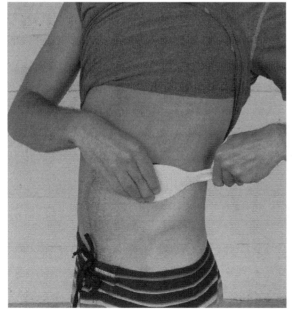

Scraping Treatment:

Not needed often. Some spots I have worked on personally are right above the pelvis bone, and mostly the external abdominal oblique (see picture for circle areas). Usually if the Quadratus Lumborum is dysfunctional, the oblique muscles will be trying to do its job of laterally stabilizing the lower back. Scraping can take care of the Quadratus Lumborum distal attachment and the External Abdominal Oblique. Also, if the Gluteus Medius is dysfunctional, this one may be trying to pick up some of the grunt work.

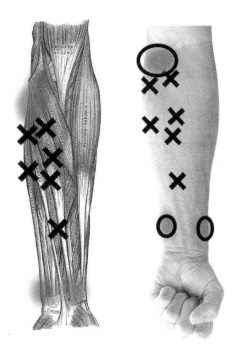

Flexor Digitorum Group/Flexor Radialis and Ulnaris

If you have hand pain, you need to take care of this muscle group. It is responsible for flexion of the wrist and hand and loves to become dysfunctional at the first signs of inflammation anywhere in the wrist.

Trigger Point Treatment:

I love using a lacrosse ball for this muscle group. Be sure to relax and shorten the muscle by making a fist and reducing the angle of the elbow joint for maximum results.

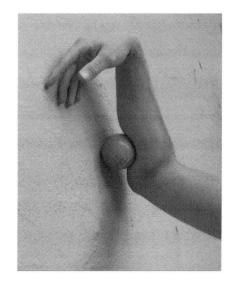

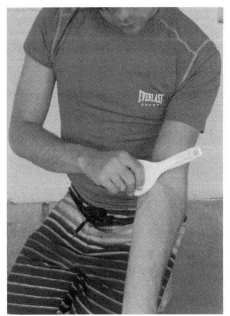

Scraping Treatment:

There are a couple of nerves to look out for, but there aren't many, so just go gently and if something does not feel right when you scrape it, do not do it. I love getting the flexor attachment point on the Medial Epicondyle. This area loves to congregate scar tissue and is easy to treat with scraping.

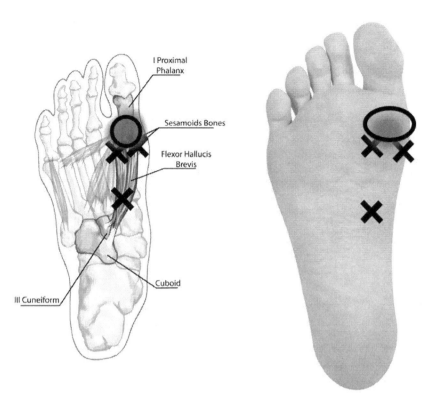

Flexor Hallucis Brevis

This is a simple muscle to treat. If you have had a bunion or foot pain, be sure to treat this one.

Trigger Point Treatment:

Roll the foot back and forth on a wooden foot roller. It is under a couple layers of muscle, and it is hard to distinguish from other foot flexor muscles, but just roll your foot over the general area that this muscle is in.

Scraping Treatment:

Scrape right behind the big toe joint. You will be hitting lots of layers of muscle if you try to scrape the whole muscle (it is pretty deep), but the area right behind the big toe joint is easy to find and important to treat with scraping.

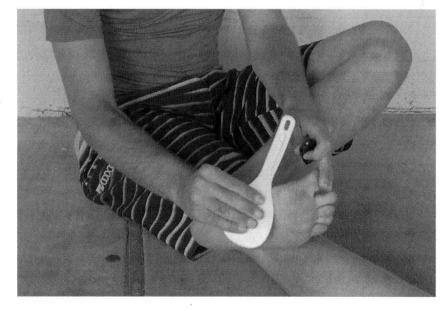

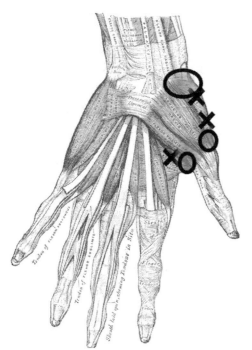

Opponens Pollicis/Adductor Pollicis

This is a very important area to treat if you have thumb pain. This muscle seems to always have a tender and treatable spot right at the base of the palm. This is the most important trigger point on this muscle group in my opinion; it is the most proximal part of the Opponens Pollicis muscle, furthest from the thumb.

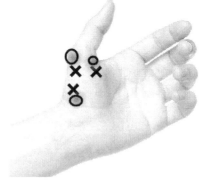

Trigger Point Treatment:

I love using a knuckle to treat this area, but what works really well is a computer mouse ball. In the old computer mice, they used to have a little ball at the bottom of the mouse. Try to find one of these and use it to roll this area out on a table. If you can't find one of these balls, use a rubber bouncy ball found next to the gumball machines in grocery stores.

Scraping Treatment:

If you have thumb pain, then I would scrape this area. If not, you probably will be just fine with the trigger point treatment. If you have a lot of dysfunction in this area, give scraping a shot.

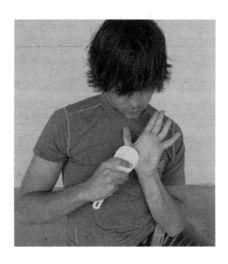

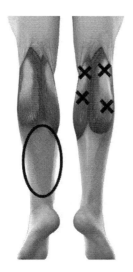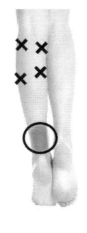

Gastrocnemius

If you have knee pain and or ankle/foot pain, you need to take care of this muscle. It crosses not only the ankle joints, but also the knee joint. This one commonly becomes dysfunctional quickly if you have Plantar Fasciitis. Luckily, it is extremely easy to get to, and you can palpate nearly the entire muscle without much effort. If you have knee issues, this muscle will become dysfunctional and later cause foot/ankle issues. If you have foot/ankle issues, this muscle will become dysfunctional and later cause knee issues. Be sure to get this thing working properly as soon as possible!

Trigger Point Treatment:

I love putting one calf muscle over the opposite legs knee and let the weight of your leg dig into the other legs Gastrocnemius muscle. You will feel where the trigger points are pretty quickly. For some people this muscle will take quite a few sessions to release most of the pain that this muscle causes, so hang in there if you do not notice much pain relief after the first couple sessions. Usually this one becomes dysfunctional slowly over a long time, so it can take a long time to release.

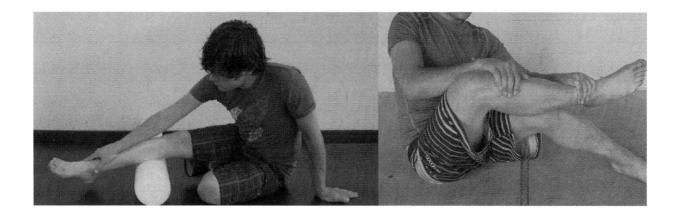

Scraping Treatment:

The Achilles tendon loves to harbor a ton of scar tissue in the sheath that encapsulates it. You should work the whole tendon, and then try going over the muscle and see if there is any grainy texture up there. Two places that are trouble causing areas are the attachment on the Calcaneus and where the Gastrocnemius attaches to the Achilles tendon.

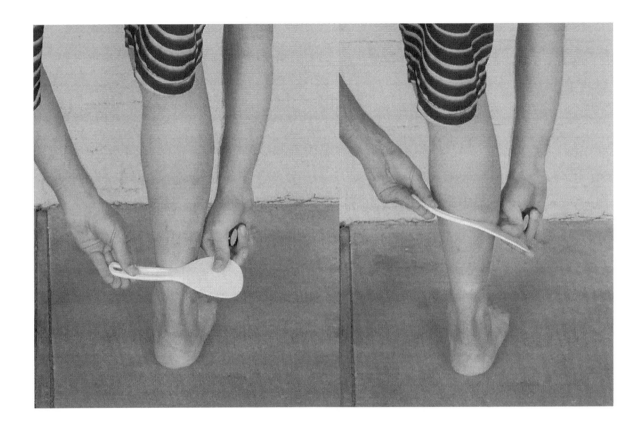

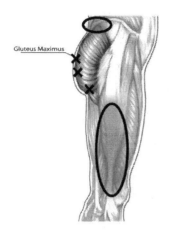

Gluteus Maximus

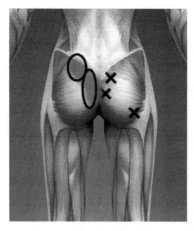

Gluteus Maximus

This is a commonly dysfunctional muscle that radiates pain to many different regions around the glutes. You must get rid of the trigger points in this muscle if you have any hip or back issues. This muscle is usually very weak in our general population because of how much time we spend seated. After you rub the trigger points out, and take care of the scraping, the kinetic chain stretches will help out a lot. This muscle is so thick and big that it will take a lot to fully release this thing and bring it back into functioning order. After three days of consistent trigger point work, this thing will be firing much more properly and will tilt your pelvis in a more favorable position. The Rectus Abdominis and Gluteus Maximus both are needed to tilt your pelvis backward (posterior pelvic tilt), and if these two muscles are weak from sitting, the pelvis will not be tilted properly (it will be in anterior pelvic tilt). When the pelvis is not situated properly, the sacrum and lower back will be at a mechanical disadvantage and instability issues will arise.

Trigger Point Treatment:
The best way to take care of this muscle: Take a lacrosse ball, put it on the ground, and roll your entire Gluteus Maximus, with your body weight, all over the muscle. You will find trigger points quickly, especially on the curve of bone where the muscle originates from (iliac crest). Roll the ball slowly and deeply into the tender tissue, and give each tender spot 6 slow strokes. After working on these trigger points for some time, you will be able to reach deep trigger points. Keep massaging this muscle out for a couple weeks and keep an eye on it. After your pain is gone, practice body weight squats a couple times a week to strengthen this muscle to prevent dysfunction from coming back.

Scraping Treatment:

This muscle is really thick, and scraping it will not help most people. Some people (myself included) will have huge knots all over the muscle. It will almost seem like the whole muscle is in spasm and causes a lot of pain. For these people, using the lacrosse ball method above will be a bit too much. For these people, they should use a foam roller first to get rid of some of the trigger points, and then use a scraping tool to hit all the circle areas as shown in the pictures. If you have knee pain, the IT band should be scraped. Remember that the IT band does not "get tight"; we scrape it so that it will not be adhered to other sheets of fascia nearby. It loves to adhere in a lot of areas, so it is best to scrape the whole IT band softly to see where the dysfunctional fascia is. The first time scraping this area will be painful, but is not so bad after you do a couple passes over the structure.

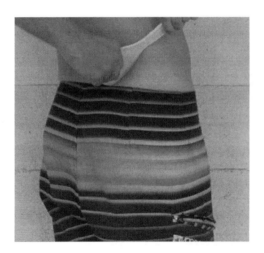

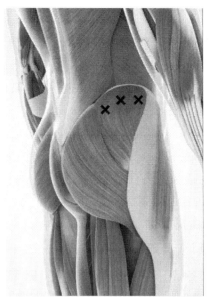

Gluteus Medius

This is a very important muscle in walking gait mechanics. This muscle shifts the weight of your body back and forth from one leg to the other.

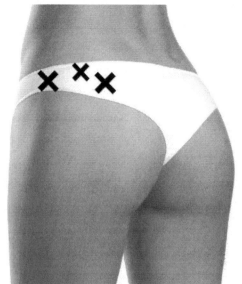

If this muscle is dysfunctional at all, the work load will be taken by the Quadtratus Lumborum. This will cause back strain and lots of pain. If this muscle is not functioning properly, then the thigh bone (femur) will not rotate and move properly, causing excessive strain on other structures, including the knee. It is a very important muscle to take care of!

Trigger Point Treatment:
Put a lacrosse ball on the floor, lay your side buttock on the ball, and slowly massage the area out. If this is much too difficult and/or sensitive, use a bigger ball or use the lacrosse ball against a wall.

Scraping Treatment:
This one will not respond to scraping treatment. It is too covered and both attachment points are hidden deep under other muscles. Some of the superior fibers can respond to scraping. See Gluteus Minimus.

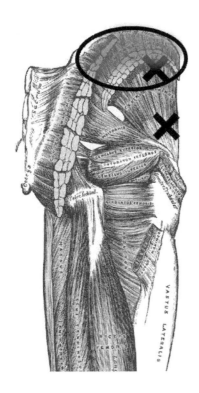

Gluteus Minimus

This is an important muscle for hip biomechanics. It is pretty deep unfortunately, and in order to treat this muscle, the Gluteus Medius must be soft and supple in order to reach it.

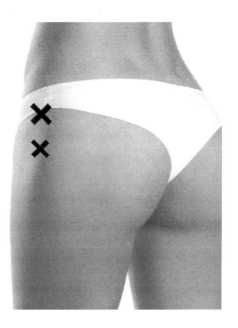

Trigger Point Treatment:

There is a very important trigger point above the head of the femur. This is its most distal attachment point. This area can send pain to many far away areas of the body. I love using a lacrosse ball to this area. After you release the Gluteus Medius, this area will become a lot easier to treat. Do slow and deep strokes with the lacrosse ball. Using the neck of the femur (thigh bone), you will find where this muscle is situated. Be sure to look carefully at the photo and where the ball is rubbing. The placement of the lacrosse ball is key for releasing this muscle.

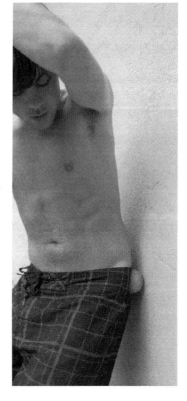

Another way to release this muscle is by putting a back buddy bar around a pole, and leaning one of the knobs into this muscle.

Scraping Treatment:

Most of this muscle is much too deep to scrape, but the superior portion can respond extremely well to scraping. It is the most superior portion of attachment for the medius and minimus.

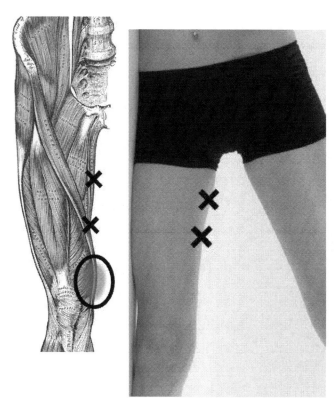

Gracilis

If you have a medial meniscus tear, this muscle will be pretty sensitive. This muscle is easily torn in certain sports and takes a long time to recover from injury. Be very careful with this area. It will be tender at first, but will respond nicely after a couple of sessions and be much easier to treat.

Trigger Point Treatment:

Big foam roller works best. Go on your hands and knees, lift one leg up and stick the foam roller under it. Your legs will be in a "frog leg" position. Try to roll all the way up the attachment point on the pelvis and down the length of both muscles. There are some nerves nearby and they cause a different feeling. Trigger point pain has a distinct feeling. If you feel a "scary" kind of pain, it is probably a nerve and you need to reduce the pressure.

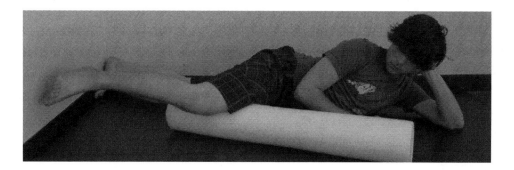

Scraping Treatment:

Be sure to go slowly at first and build up pressure slowly. This muscle crosses not only the hip joint, but also the knee joint. Be sure to treat the tendon all the way down to the tibia (shin bone).

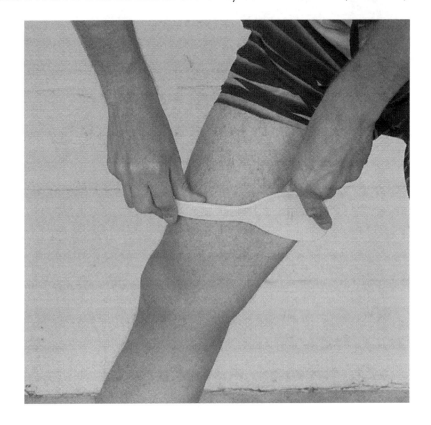

Infraspinatus

If you have pain in the front of your shoulder, you will have dysfunction in this muscle. This little muscle has to do a lot of

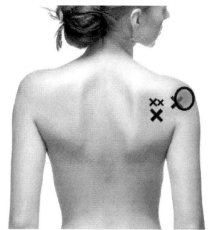

Rotator Cuff Muscles

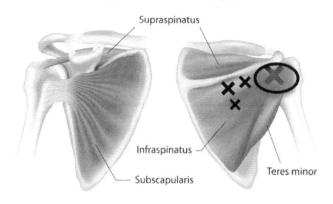

Supraspinatus

Infraspinatus

Subscapularis

Teres minor

Anterior view   Posterior view

work to stabilize the unstable shoulder. It is one of the few muscles that externally rotate the shoulder, so it loves to become dysfunctional quickly. If you have any shoulder issues for that matter, this one is a prime suspect for dysfunction.

Trigger Point Treatment:

Back buddy stick is a great tool to get rid of dysfunction in this muscle. Another great tool is a lacrosse ball against a wall.

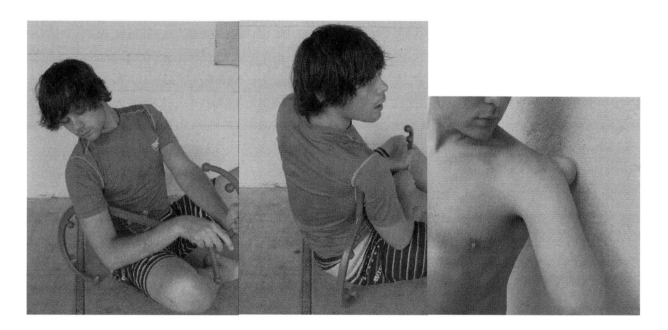

Scraping Treatment:

This is one of the few muscles that you must have someone else scrape. It is nearly impossible to do it to yourself. You want to lay on a bed, on your stomach, with your arm hanging off the side. Look at the photos carefully and notice where the muscle is located. Use the spine of the scapula to reference where it is located – the muscle is just below the scapulas spine (the bony protrusion on your shoulder blade). Scrape the whole muscle, especially the attachment to the arm (humorous) area. A small convex tool works best. Scrape right behind the shoulder joint, on the Infraspinatus tendon, and you may find some nodules of scar tissue.

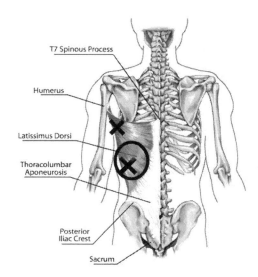

T7 Spinous Process
Humerus
Latissimus Dorsi
Thoracolumbar Aponeurosis
Posterior Iliac Crest
Sacrum

Latissimus Dorsi

This is a big muscle! It connects to the lower back and goes up the side of the body and attaches to the front of the humorous bone. This muscle crosses many joints, so it can cause some widespread issues if it is dysfunctional. This muscle is pretty thin and covers a lot of area. I find the kinetic chain stretches for this muscle really effective at treating dysfunction.

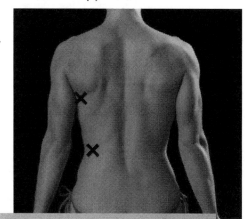

Trigger Point Treatment:

Using a big foam roller, rub the side of your back, where the Latissimus Dorsi is located. I usually do not find specific trigger points in this muscle; instead I find that the whole muscle becomes a little tender. I like to massage the whole muscle out gently with the foam roller which seems to do the trick.

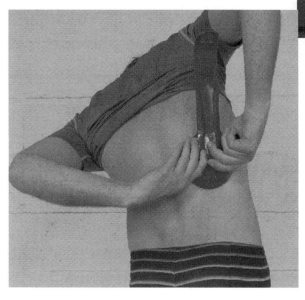

Scraping Treatment:

You can scrape at the lower attachment and over the belly of the muscle if it has been dysfunctional for many months (especially after a shoulder surgery that required being immobilized for months on end in a sling). If not, you can get by with a little trigger point work, then move straight to the kinetic chain stretches for this muscle.

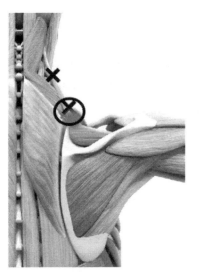
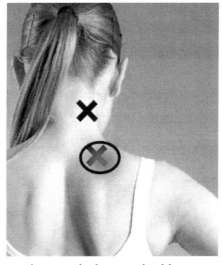

Levator Scapulae

If you have an office job and sit hunched over a computer, this muscle will be dysfunctional and tender. Of all the muscles, I find that this muscle, the Trapezius, and the Vastus Lateralis always have a trigger point. This is because they have to pull bones in varying directions all the time. The distal attachment for this muscle, into the scapula, loves to build up scar tissue around the muscle and around nearby structures. The scraping methods for this muscle are extremely effective, and once you experience relief from pain after releasing this muscle and its associated fascia, you will keep an eye on it forever.

Trigger Point Treatment:

Rub this thing out with a back buddy stick or with lacrosse ball against a wall. It feels really good to rub this muscle out.

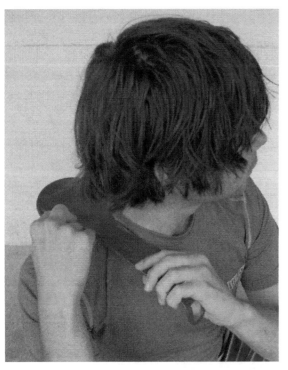

Scraping Treatment:

Take a flat or concave edge tool and rub the entire length of the muscle. It is much easier to have someone do it for you. Also try scraping the area where it attaches into the scapula. Unlike the photo, use lubrication and run the tool over your bare skin!

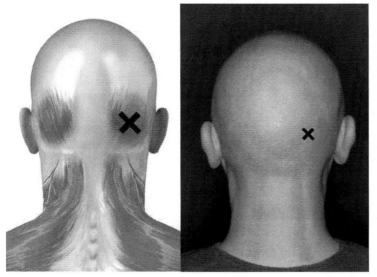

Occipitalis

If you have headaches, this muscle, along with the Sternocleidomastoid, will probably be dysfunctional. If you have had hamstring, back muscle, or neck issues from sitting in a desk all day, the dysfunction can sneak its way up to this muscle because they all belong to the same kinetic chain. It is easy to work out the trigger points, but do not scrape this muscle for most people have hair in this area!

Trigger Point Treatment:

Use lacrosse balls or a small foam roller on the ground to work the tension out of this muscle. Some will find extremely tender spots in this muscle if they have had long standing issues with neck pain/headaches etc.

Scraping Treatment:

Not recommended. If you have a shaved head and this muscle seems to keep getting trigger points consistently, then give scraping a shot. Most will be fine with just trigger point work.

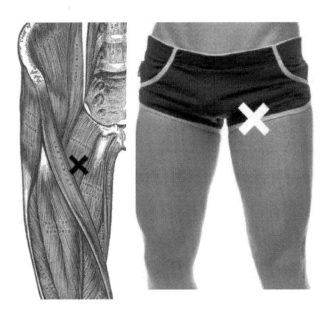

Pectineus

This hard to reach muscle is very important to treat trigger points if you have hip pain.

Trigger Point Treatment:

Lay on the ground with a big foam roller under your upper/front thigh. Slowly roll out the area where the Pectineus lies. Nearby nerves will make it difficult at times to get to the muscle. If you feel anything too sensitive, ease up on the pressure. Be sure to massage really high up on the thigh in order to hit this muscle.

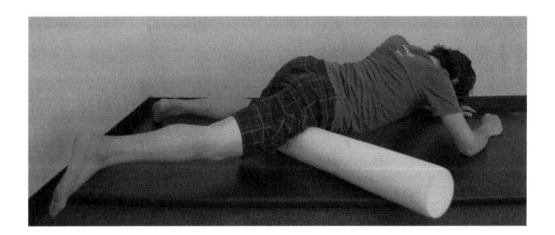

Scraping Treatment:

Not recommended due to nerves/lymphatic structures in this area.

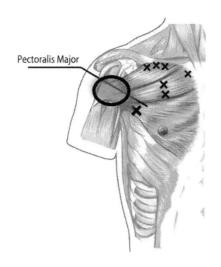 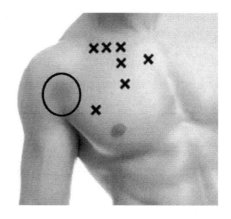

Pectoralis Major

This muscle is very commonly dysfunctional in anterior shoulder pain cases. If you have shoulder pain, check this whole muscle for dysfunction. This thing can cause tons of pain in the shoulder if you have trigger points anywhere inside this muscle.

Trigger Point Treatment:
Use a lacrosse ball against a wall. Most important thing to do here is to check every part of the muscle. There are fibers that extend up to the clavicle and sternum. You must check every area out.

Scraping Treatment:
Only scrape the area indicated in the picture. Make sure that the arm is in the proper position to scrape the area properly. Use a big convex tool to scrape the area.

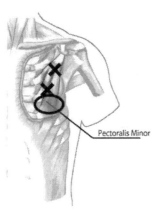

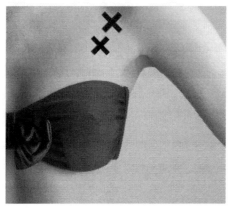

Pectoralis Minor

Pectoralis Minor

This is a very important muscle for scapular stability. If you are in a desk hunched over a computer all day, this muscle will be shortened and tender. Luckily, it is easy to treat and responds well to trigger point treatment.

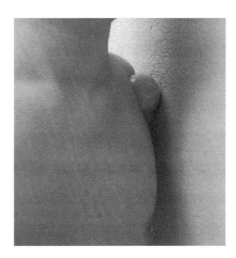

Trigger Point Treatment:
Use a lacrosse ball against a wall to treat this muscle's trigger points. In order to get deep into the muscle, move your shoulder forward and backward (protraction/retraction) while pushing the lacrosse ball into the muscle. This will make the treatment much more effective.

Scraping Treatment:
There is only a small portion of the muscle that can be treated with scraping. The reason is because most of the muscle is very deep and hard to get to, and because adhesions love to appear between the Pectoralis Minor and the Pectoralis Major. Running over the area where they run by each other is sufficient enough to break up the adhesions. Use a convex tool to go in deep.

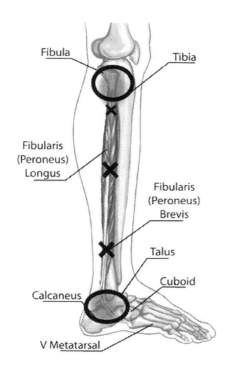

Fibula

Tibia

Fibularis (Peroneus) Longus

Fibularis (Peroneus) Brevis

Talus

Cuboid

Calcaneus

V Metatarsal

Peroneal Group

This muscle group is responsible for eversion of the foot and ankle. If it is dysfunctional and shortened, the foot will be susceptible to over pronation due to the excessive eversion. Pronation is very important to have because it absorbs shock from the ground. If the foot is not moving, and is held in a static position, unable to absorb shock from the ground, problems can arise VERY quickly. This muscle group is located on the outside of the calf muscles.

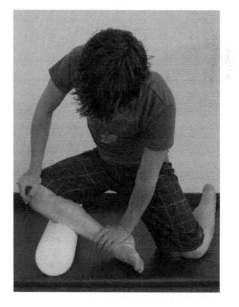

Trigger Point Treatment:

I love using a lacrosse ball or small foam roller for this area. The best method I have ever found is to use a stainless steel water bottle, fill it up with hot water, and roll this muscle out. Lie down on your side, with your legs bent, and slowly roll the water bottle over these muscles.

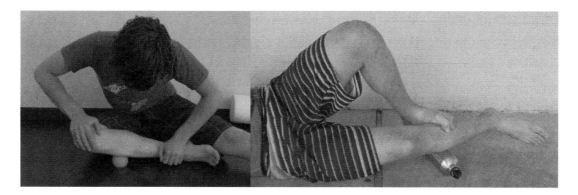

Scraping Treatment:

Scraping is really effective for this muscle, but you must be careful of the nerve that passes next to this muscle on the upper portion of the muscle. Try scraping the tendons and thicker portions of the muscle. If you have any kind of outside ankle pain, or outer foot pain (near the pinky toe), this scraping will give you a lot of pain relief. Use a convex tool of any size. It is easy to reach and easy to scrape.

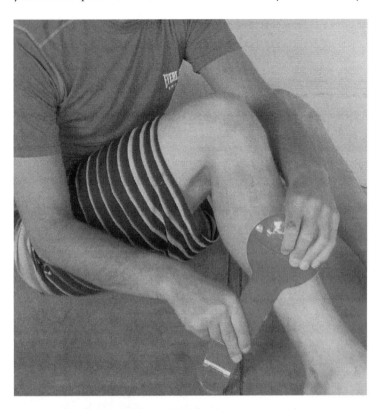

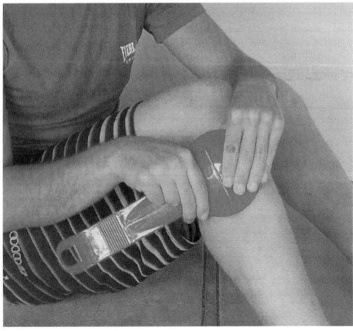

Piriformis

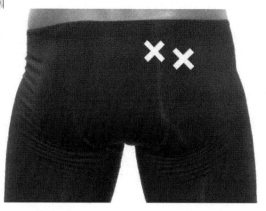

This is a deep external rotator of the hip. It is one of the most commonly dysfunctional muscles in the body and directly causes a condition called sciatica. If this muscle is harboring trigger points or dysfunctional fascia, it can cause all sorts of pain down the side and back of the leg.

Trigger Point Treatment:
Lacrosse ball is the most effective. Lie down on your knees up, and push a lacrosse back, with your ball into this muscle. Massage the whole length of the muscle, but be careful about going too low. This is because the sciatic nerve passes right under the Piriformis muscle. Static and slow rubbing motions work well on this muscle.

Scraping Treatment:
Scraping is hard to do because of this muscle's location under Gluteal muscles, but it is possible. All you need to do is know exactly where the muscle is (use bony landmarks nearby), and use a medium sized convex tool. If there are any trigger points or dysfunctional fascia in the Gluteus Maximus, you will not be able to reach this muscle. Work on that muscle first, and then come back to the Piriformis.

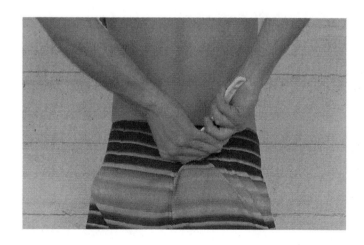

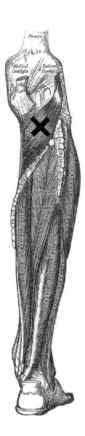

Popliteus

This muscle controls the rotation of the knee. If you have knee pain, this muscle will probably be in a light spasm. It is close to nerves, so look at the pictures closely to find the trigger points.

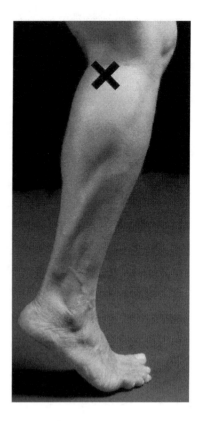

Trigger Point Treatment:

I love shoving a lacrosse ball behind my knee joint and closing my knee joint around the ball with my arms. Besides this method, use your hands. It is a sensitive spot and does not require too much pressure to release this muscle.

Scraping Treatment:

Do not scrape this muscle.

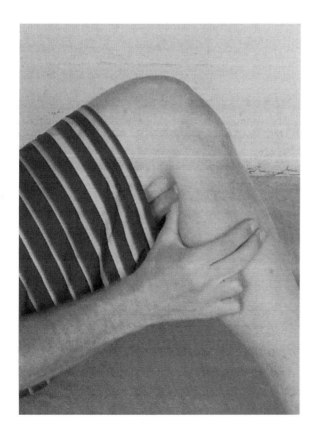

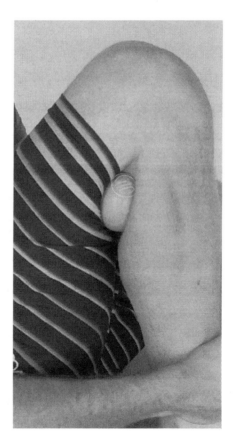

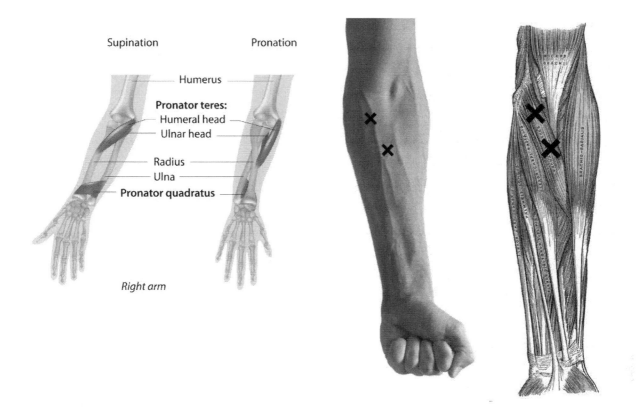

Pronator Teres

This muscle is a primary mover when it comes to forearm rotation. It can be shortened if you type at a desk for more than a couple hours a day. If you have a manual labor job, such as wrenching, this muscle can become overworked. Loosening screws with a screwdriver put this muscle into overdrive, and if done every day for months, it can cause issues.

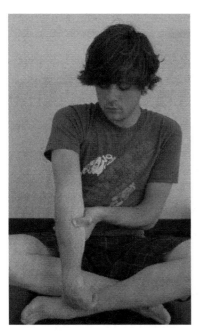

Trigger Point Treatment:
I like to use a form of dynamic release. Find the muscle by contracting it (by pronating the forearm). You will feel it as a taught band in the forearm in the area in the picture above. Then you want to feel the length of the muscle and try to find tender spots. When you find the tender spots, keep your thumb on the area. Then, flex the elbow and wrist while pronating and apply pressure to tender spot. Next, slowly extend the elbow and wrist and supinate the forearm all at the same time. A video is available of me explaining how to do this at http://www.mstrtherapy.com.

First, find the pronater teres by pronating the forearm. Feel the muscle for tender spots.

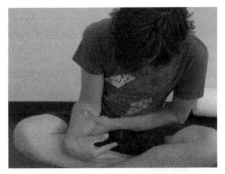

Second, keep thumb on pronator teres and flex the wrist and elbow, then apply pressure with your thumb on tender spot.

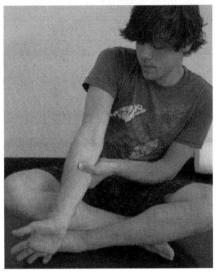

Third, while applying pressure to tender spot, extend elbow and wrist and supinate at the same time.

Scraping Treatment:
This muscle is too deep to scrape, but the area around it can be scraped. Sometimes you can use a convex tool to reach deep trigger points. Instead of scraping, use the tool to rub back and forth on deep trigger points. There are no specific areas; just feel for tender spots and treat accordingly.

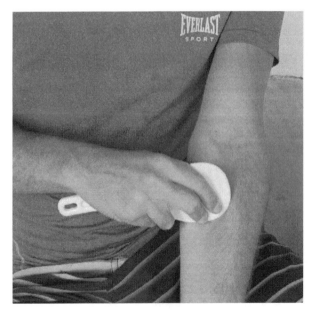

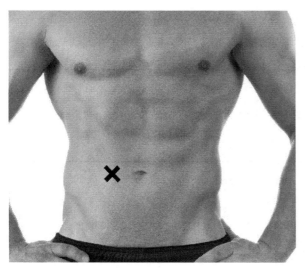

Psoas Group

This is an extremely important muscle for back pain and hip pain. Most people today love to sit down. They sit in cars to and from work, they sit all day at work, then when they come home they sit on their couch. It is no surprise that these people's Psoas muscles are extremely dysfunctional. The body says, "So you like to sit down and shorten your Psoas? Ok then, I will make this muscle dreadfully short!" The problem with this is that the Psoas should not be shortened. It needs to be able to lengthen to stabilize the pelvis and lower back. Nearly every person with back pain or hip pain will have some degree of dysfunction in this muscle, and it needs to be treated. Even people that do not have pain, but sit down all day, will have some form of dysfunction in this muscle. It is very important to treat, but somewhat difficult to do so. Long-term functionality of this muscle can be achieved with kinetic chain stretches and better ergonomics. Its best to walk around every half an hour at work than it is to buy an expensive ergonomic chair, however. Be sure to not sit for too long after you treat this muscle, especially if you do not want its dysfunctional characteristics to come back.

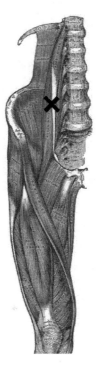

Trigger Point Treatment:

If you are skinny or healthy without too much abdominal fat, this muscle can be felt with your own hands. Lay on the ground, on your back with your knees bent at 90 degree angles and your feet flat on the ground. Put one hand's finger's 1 inch to either side of your belly button and push this hand into your stomach slowly with your other hand. Or, you can use the supported finger technique in the picture below. You should feel a hot dog shaped object just under the skin. Next, move both knees close to each other, then further from each other. This should treat the trigger point spasm pretty nicely.

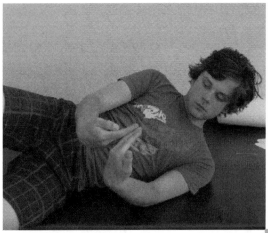

Supported Finger Technique

Find the muscle by pushing in 1 inch lateral (lateral means away from the bodies midline) to the belly button on either side. Feel for hot dog shape and press into the muscle.

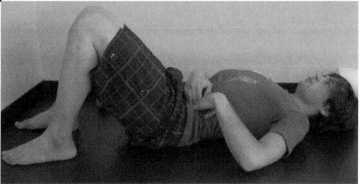

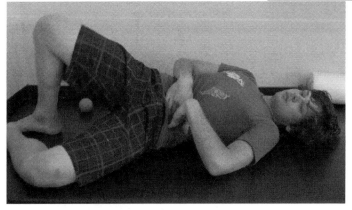

Then, relax leg on side being treated and let it slowly fall to the ground. Then while still applying pressure to muscle, bring leg up to the beginning position, and then repeat.

Scraping Treatment:

Impossible to scrape.

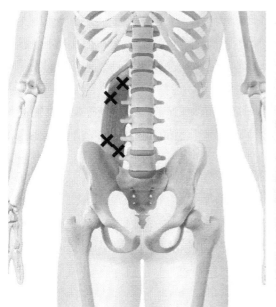 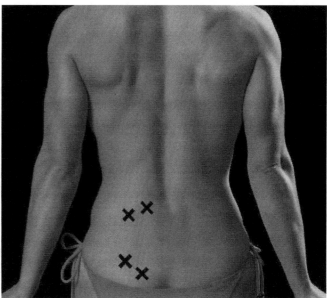

Quadratus Lumborum

This is a very important muscle in the treatment of chronic lower back pain. If abnormal walking gait is suspected because of Gluteus Medius weakness, this muscle becomes overworked and later on dysfunctional, causing lots of lower back pain. It is responsible for lateral and twisting movements. If trigger points in this muscle are severe, everything hurts to do. Lots of pain everywhere!

Trigger Point Treatment:
This muscle has deep trigger points. You need to come from the sides of the back to reach this muscle because the back muscles cover a good majority of the palpable area of this muscle. This means you need to angle the pressure so that the pressure goes in and towards the midline of the body. Use a back buddy stick or lacrosse ball. Having a professional trigger point therapist can be helpful if this muscle is severely dysfunctional. It can be hard to find the trigger points, but a professional can find them pretty quickly.

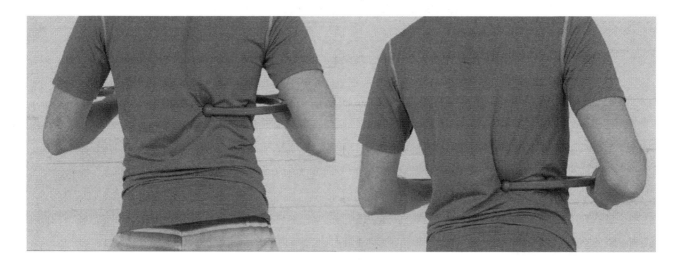

Scraping Treatment:

Outer edges can be scraped. Use a convex tool of any size. If you have excess body fat, these areas can be extremely hard to treat with scraping tools.

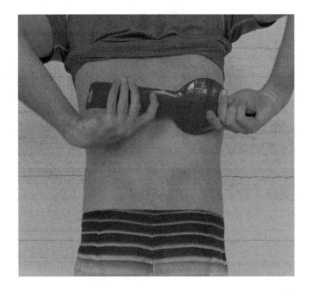

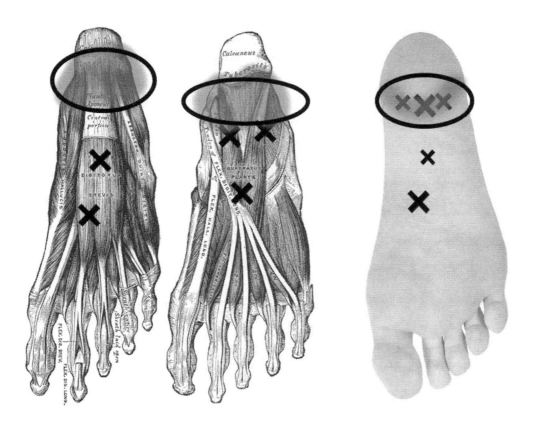

Quadratus Plantae and Other Deep Foot Flexors

If you have foot pain, release this area. It can directly cause plantar fasciitis pain symptoms and more.

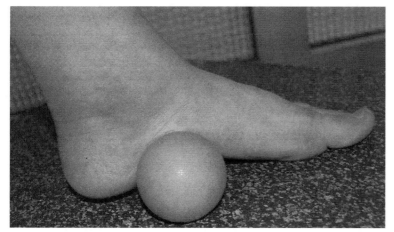

Trigger Point Treatment:
Use a foot roller or lacrosse ball. Roll the whole foot out, including inside and outside edges. Wooden foot roller is most ideal, but you can use a lacrosse ball.

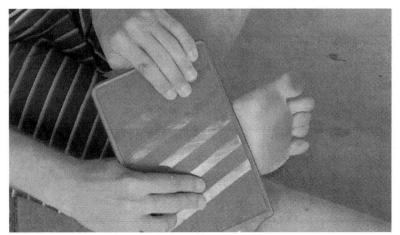

Scraping Treatment:
Use a big straight edge tool to scrape this area. Scrape the whole area. Will be painful at first, go slow and build up pressure. (sorry for the dirty feet!)

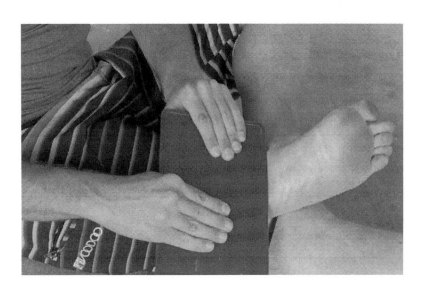

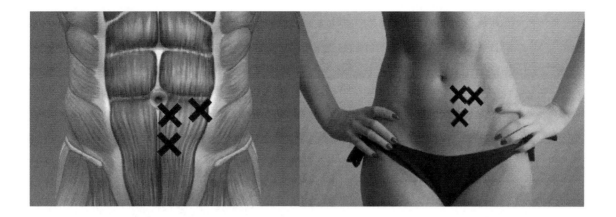

Rectus Abdominis

This muscle loves to become weak from having anterior pelvic tilt (what most sedentary people have). It needs to be treated and strengthened along with the Gluteal muscles so that your pelvis is more stable. If you have had any recent abdominal surgery, this muscle may be in a spasm state.

Trigger Point Treatment:
Use hands to massage out trigger points. If you have a big ball to roll your stomach on, that works well too.

Scraping Treatment:
Not usually needed. Trigger point therapy takes care of most issues. The only time it is needed is over an old scar. If you have a huge scar from a surgery in this area, and it has been closed for some time (at least 4-5 months), you can scrape the area to make the area strong and functional. After surgery, the skin on top of a scar can become tacked down to underlying structures. When you first start to scrape a scar, go slow and be gentle. It does take a long time for the scar tissue to rearrange and remodel itself. After a while of scraping treatments, pinch the skin on the scar to see how tacked down it is. If it is more supple and soft and does not adhere to the structures under the skin, you are doing a good job.

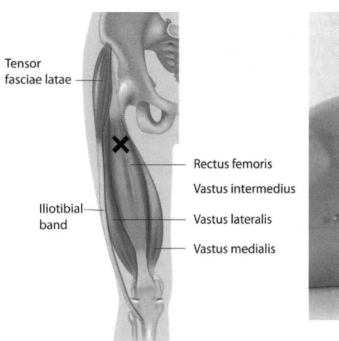

Tensor
fasciae latae

Iliotibial
band

Rectus femoris

Vastus intermedius

Vastus lateralis

Vastus medialis

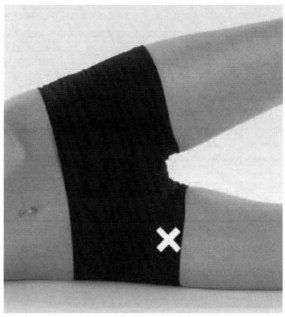

Rectus Femoris

This is a very important muscle for knee pain and hip pain. It is a multiple joint muscle and is prone to dysfunction. If you sit down all day long, this muscle will probably be shortened.

Trigger Point Treatment:
I love using a rolling pin to treat this muscle. Other options are foam rollers. The Rectus Femoris is an easy muscle to massage and it feels good to treat the trigger points.

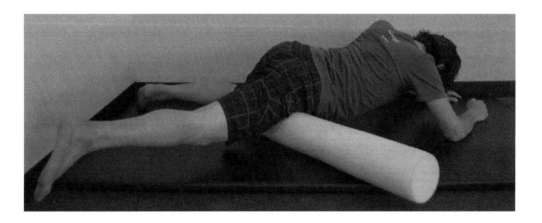

Scraping Treatment:

Attachment areas are common spots for scar tissue to form. Use a large concave or straight edge tool.

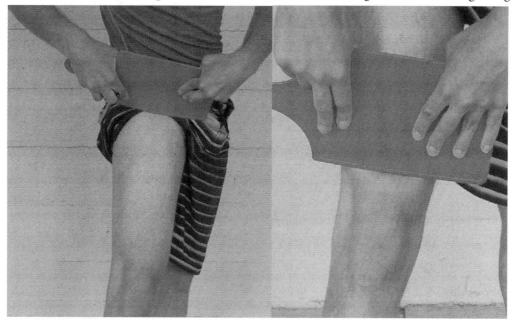

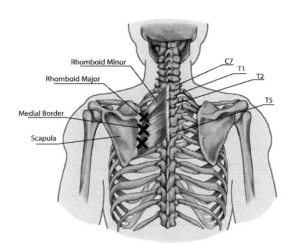

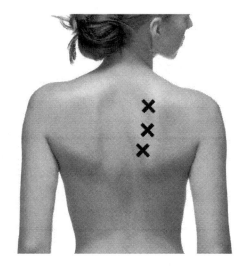

Rhomboid

This muscle lifts the shoulder blades and retracts them towards the back. Is usually weak in the general population and is usually lengthened more than needed due to people being hunched over desks.

Trigger Point Treatment:

There are many ways to fix this muscle. You can use a foam roller over the mid back area and lacrosse balls on the mid-back. I actually love to buy those shiatsu massage chairs at Costco to rub this muscles trigger points out.

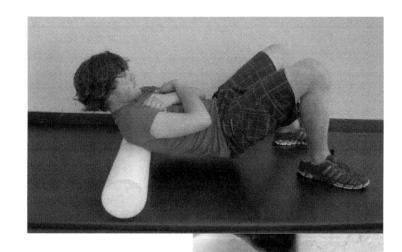

Also, the classic lacrosse ball against the wall technique.

Scraping Treatment:

This muscle is too deep to scrape. Focus on trigger point work.

Sartorius

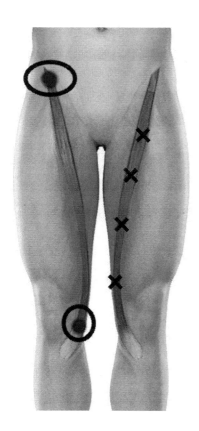

This muscle has a very interesting shape and function. This muscle wraps across the thigh and passes over the hip joint and the knee joint. This muscle rotates the knee and hip and is needed for proper walking gait dynamics. If you prefer to sit with one leg over the other, that leg that you cross over may have a shortened Sartorius.

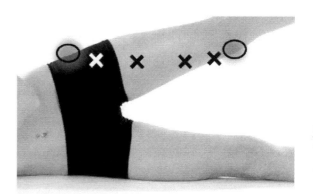

Trigger Point Treatment:
Cross one leg over the other leg so that you can shorten the Sartorius. Feel the whole muscle for trigger points with your hands. They can be anywhere in the muscle, but I usually find them near the proximal insertion, near the Tensor Fascia Latae. Use a fist to massage out the trigger point.

Scraping Treatment:
The insertions respond well to scraping treatment, but not the muscles belly so much.

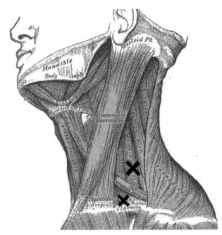 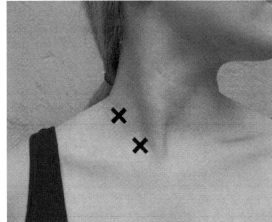

Scalene Group

This is a tricky muscle group. It can cause pain far away from the muscle, including the hand and shoulder. I personally had so much pain from this muscle alone after my last shoulder surgery, and if left untreated, can make you have 24/7 pain in your shoulder and hand. Muscle dysfunction can also cause nerve entrapment due to the nerve bundle that passes through this muscle group.

Trigger Point Treatment:

What you need to do to get to this muscle is feel for the Sternocleidomastoid muscle. Once you find its attachment on the Sternum, move it out of the way with your hand (move it towards your throat) and right under this muscle lies the Anterior Scalene. Slowly massage it out. If you hit a nerve, it will be painful. If you go slowly and carefully, you should not hit any nerves. The nerves feel like ropes next to the muscles. Just feel around for muscle knots and they should be pretty obvious when you hit them. Use your fingers to slowly massage them out.

The Posterior Scalene and Middle Scalene can be massaged by having someone push an elbow into this area. You can also massage it yourself with your hands, but it can be very difficult. Watch out for the nerve that passes next to the Middle Scalene muscle.

If this is at all confusing to you, check out http://www.mstrtherapy.com for a video on how to treat this muscle. You can find it under the treatment video section under neck pain.

Scraping Treatment:

Do not scrape this muscle.

Semitendinosus/Semimembranosus

This muscle is responsible for knee stability through knee rotation and fine-tuned flexion. It moves the hip and knee joints. It is prone to

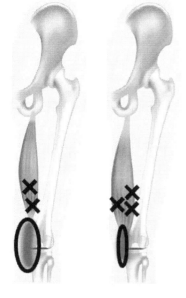

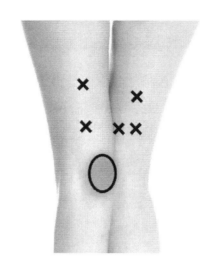

dysfunction in people who spend their days sitting in chairs. If dysfunctional, it puts the pelvis in an unstable position and can directly cause lower back pain.

Semitendinosus   Semimembranosus

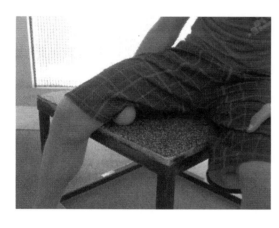

Trigger Point Treatment:
Use two lacrosse balls on a flat bench to roll out any trigger points you find. This is a big muscle and to find the trigger points requires some patience. Watch out for the Sciatic nerve near the origin insertion on the upper portion of the muscle. It is very sensitive and painful if you hit the Sciatic nerve with a lacrosse ball. Try to stay in the belly of the muscle.

You can also use a small foam roller to roll out these muscles if they are too sensitive to be worked out with the lacrosse balls.

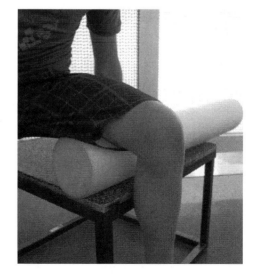

Scraping Treatment:

Scrape the whole muscle. It will feel gritty if you have hip or knee issues. Try to scrape the outside area of the muscle and you should find lots of scar tissue built up. Use a big straight edge tool to scrape this area out.

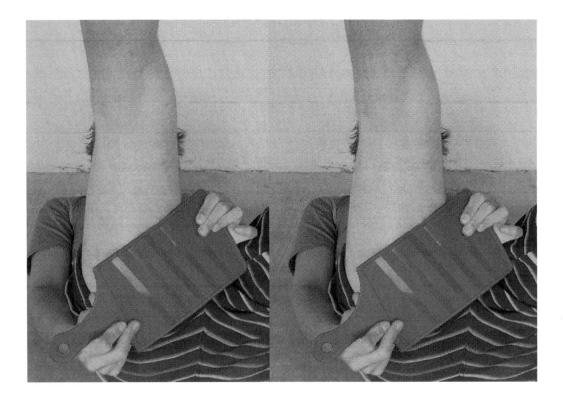

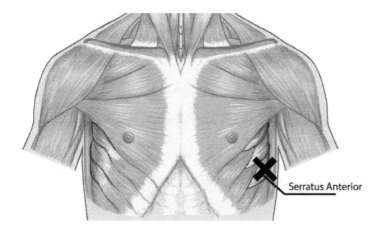

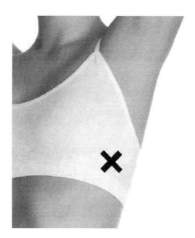

Serratus Anterior

Serratus Anterior

This is an extremely important scapula stabilizer and also assists in breathing. When this muscle is dysfunctional, it can hurt to breathe. If you have to expel air out of the lungs fast, such as sneezing or coughing, this muscle will shoot pain all over your sides and mid back. It is responsible for protracting your scapula and in most people it will be inhibited or weak.

Trigger Point Treatment:
Wrap your arm around your side and feel this muscles location for its main trigger point. It may take a second of feeling around, but when you find this trigger point, you will know it. It is usually pretty sensitive and feels really good to massage out.

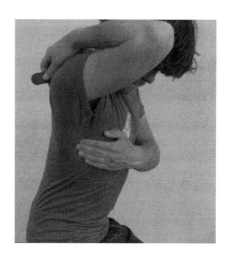

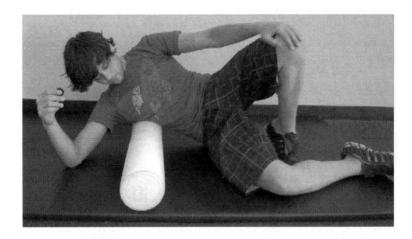

You can also lie on a foam roller and massage this area out. Should be a big foam roller and you should not over arch your back when you lay on it.

Scraping Treatment:

Too many exposed and sensitive ribs nearby makes this muscle treatable only by trigger point massage. Some argue that you can scrape the muscle's belly, but it is better if you just stick with trigger point massage here.

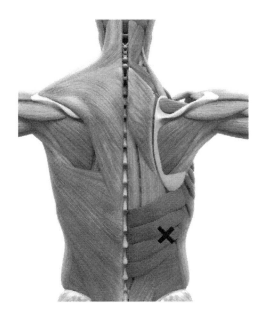
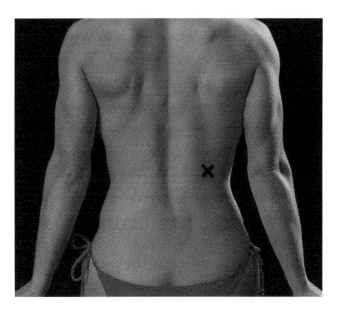

Serratus Posterior Inferior

This is a very important muscle for twisting movements of the spine and forced expiration. Because it is a breathing muscle, it is very important to make sure all the dysfunction is taken care of for proper breathing mechanics.

Trigger Point Treatment:
This muscle responds well to a lacrosse ball against the wall and The Back Buddy © stick. This muscle is one muscle that is more effectively dealt with by having someone else rub it out. Lie on your stomach, on a bed and have someone find its main trigger point. Have them slowly rub an aggressive trigger point tool into it, such as a Knobble©. Once they hit the trigger point, it may make you want to cry. It hurts like crazy, but eases up pretty fast.

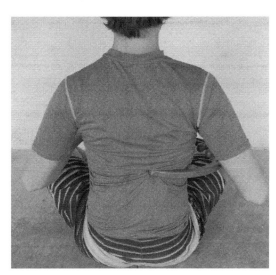

Scraping Treatment:
This deep muscle is close to ribs, so somewhat hard to isolate for scraping treatment. If you have mid back pain, try scraping the whole area.

Serratus Posterior Superior

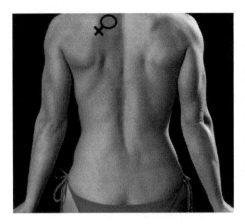

This is an important muscle due to the fact that you need it for proper breathing mechanics. This muscle lifts the ribs and expands your rib cage to let more air in your lungs. If it is dysfunctional, you are not going to be breathing as well as you should (to full capacity). It can cause a lot of upper back and hand pain if dysfunctional.

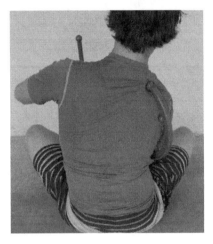

Trigger Point Treatment:

In order to reach it, you need to release the Rhomboid muscles and Trapezius first, and then move the scapula out of the way by protracting your shoulder forward, then massage the area where it is located. Use a lacrosse ball against a wall or back buddy stick to reach this muscle. It is a bit deep and in order to reach it you need to relax and let the tool sink under the skin.

Scraping Treatment:

This muscle is too deep to scrape. But you can use the scraping tool as a trigger point tool. Just press a small convex shaped tool deep into the area where this muscle is located, poke around until you find a trigger point, press the tool into the trigger point and instead of scraping, rub the trigger point out. You can use this on other deep muscles that are too deep to scrape.

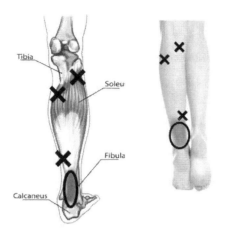

Soleus

Even though this calf muscle is a single joint muscle, it can cause quite a lot of problems. Its pain referral patterns are pretty widespread and if the trigger points in this muscle are active, you will be in a lot of pain. This is an extremely important muscle to treat if you have plantar fasciitis.

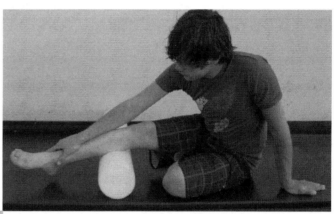

Trigger Point Treatment:
Use a rolling pin to roll out the trigger points in this muscle. Rub the opposite legs knee into this muscle while seated or use a foam roller as seen in picture below.

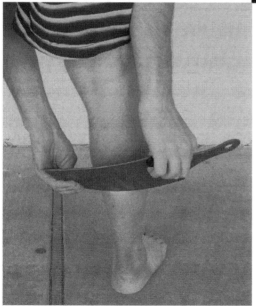

Scraping Treatment:
Tendon and inside portion is treatable with scraping treatment. Achilles tendon should also be worked out with long and slow scrapes with a big straight edge tool.

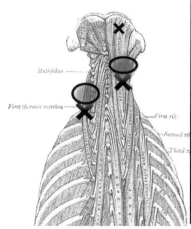 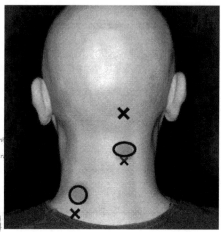

Splenius Capitis/Splenius Cervicis/Semispinalis Capitis

These three muscles are hard to distinguish from each other because they are so close to one another. I like to treat them as one "group" of muscles. They form the rear neck muscles. They can become dysfunctional from being hunched over a desk or from experiencing whip lash in a car accident.

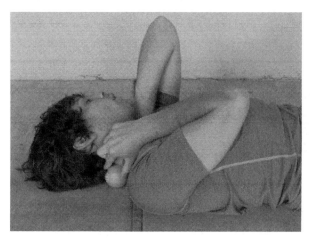

Trigger Point Treatment:

Lay on the ground with two lacrosse balls in the back of your neck. Slowly move your head on the balls until you find tender spots.

A Back Buddy Stick is also extremely useful for working out these muscles.

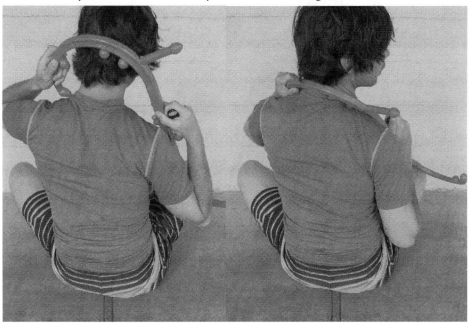

Scraping Treatment:

Scrape the whole neck up to the hair line. Start with slow strokes and build up pressure. This muscle feels great after being scraped, but it needs to be done slowly at first to see good results. Once the area "feels good", then apply more pressure. It should not be too discomforting if you go slow and steady at first.

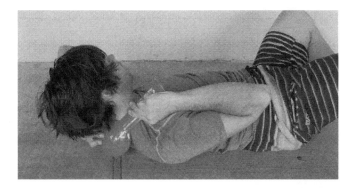

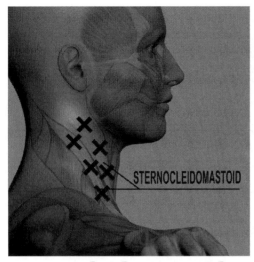 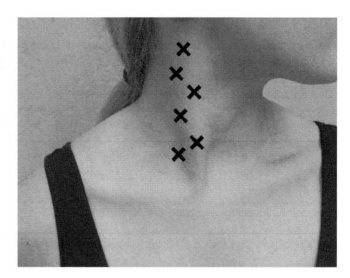

Sternocleidomastoid

If you have had headaches or neck pain, you need to rub this muscle out today! The trigger points in this muscle can cause extreme amounts of widespread pain that can last for months. It is tricky to massage at first, but when you get it down, you will be checking this muscle out every time you have neck pain and/or headache.

This muscle controls rotation of the head on its axis. It also does flexion of the neck, but extension of the head and it crosses A LOT of joints, so it is very prone to dysfunction.

Trigger Point Treatment:
Look at the pictures and notice where the muscle starts near the chest. Feel this area with your hands and find the insertion point. Gently grab the muscle starting at the bottom, and lift it off the neck ever so slightly so that you can feel the entire width of the muscle. Slowly make your way up towards the back of your head, feeling for tender spots. Trigger points can be found anywhere in this muscle, so be sure to check the whole thing out!

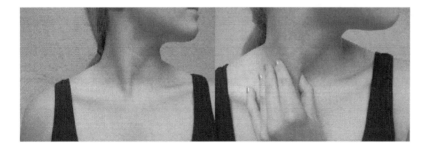

Scraping Treatment:

Scraping is possible, but only for professionals. The amount of nerves, blood vessels, and lymphatic activity that is present near this muscle makes it dangerous to scrape unless you know what you're doing. Plus, trigger point therapy works extremely well on this muscle. The only location on this muscle that I scrape is where it attaches at the base of the skull. But again, let a professional do it.

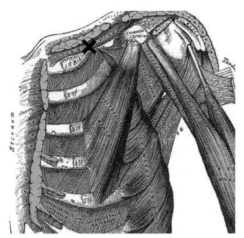

Subclavius

This is a small muscle, but it can cause a lot of pain. Luckily, it is very easy to treat.

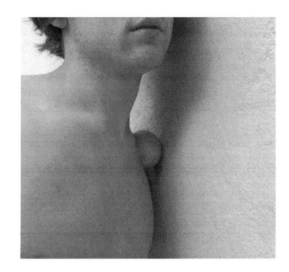

Trigger Point Treatment:

Simply use a lacrosse ball against a wall. Lift up your shoulder and push the ball under your Clavicle (collarbone). Slowly push the ball into the muscle and let your shoulder hang down. Relax and push the ball into the trigger points.

Scraping Treatment:

Not needed. There are many nerves nearby, and it responds extremely well to lacrosse ball massage.

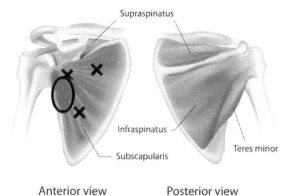

Rotator Cuff Muscles

Supraspinatus

Infraspinatus

Subscapularis

Teres minor

Anterior view   Posterior view

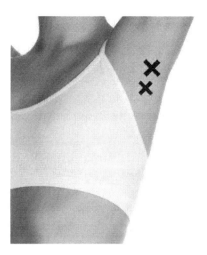

Subscapularis

This is a very important muscle if you have shoulder pain, especially if your shoulder pain is caused by instability of the shoulder joint. If you have torn your labrum (which I have personally done twice), this muscle will be EXTREMELY dysfunctional and can take some consistent effort to make it healthy again.

Trigger Point Treatment:
Using various poles, including the small poles with rounded ends on The Back Buddy © stick, works really well to get this muscle working properly again. The trigger points are very near to nerves, so if you feel a pain that is not a trigger point pain, do not push on the area. These are usually very superior and near the shoulder joint (Subscapular nerve diverges from the posterior division of the Brachial Plexus). There are many trigger points at the bottom of the muscle (inferior aspect near inferior angle of Scapula, anterior aspect).

This muscle is really hard to massage properly. Just imagine that it is in the back wall of the armpit. It is literally under the scapula.

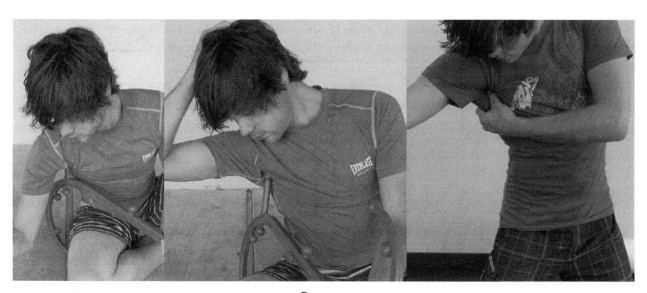

Scraping Treatment:

Scraping is important for treatment, but hard to do alone. It is much better if you have someone else do it for you. I suggest going to a Graston ® therapist for this part because it is pretty difficult. If you are brave and understand where the nerves are, then give it a shot. Try to find creative ways to be able to scrape the muscle, but while it is relaxed and lengthened.

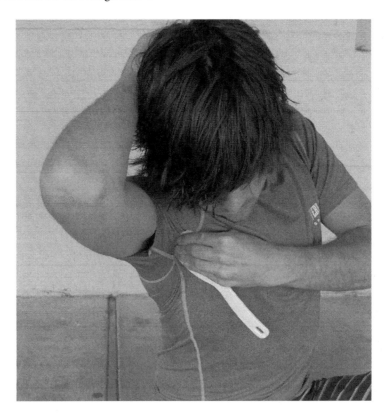

Rotator Cuff Muscles

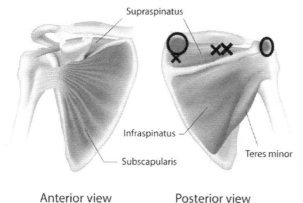

Supraspinatus

Infraspinatus

Subscapularis

Teres minor

Anterior view   Posterior view

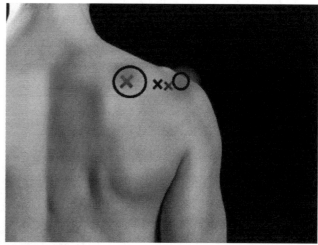

Supraspinatus

This muscle is very prone to damage due to its small size and lack of space for growth. This muscle has to travel inside a very small hole and out into the shoulder joint. When its tendon becomes inflamed, it will press on structures around it, creating pressure.

This muscle is the most commonly torn muscle of all the rotator cuff muscles and a prime mover when it comes to raising your arms to the side (Abduction).

Trigger Point Treatment:
This is hard to do properly. This muscle is somewhat deep and lies under the Trapezius. In order to treat, just push straight into it. I find that it helps to have someone dig their elbow into this muscle while you are lying down. If you can't find someone to do that, use a back buddy stick. Lacrosse balls work if you are a big and tall person, but hard to lean against a wall. I suggest trying to get someone to dig their elbow in more than anything because it is so effective.

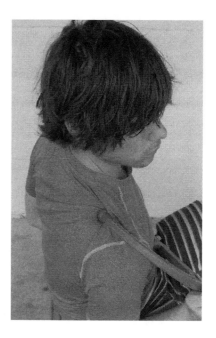

Use the spine of the scapula to reference (long bony bump that goes across your scapula and goes toward your shoulder joint) and massage right above it. There is a little canyon just above the spine of the scapula and this is where the Supraspinatus is.

Scraping Treatment:

You can scrape the Trapezius which lies on top of this muscle, and almost get into this area, but pretty difficult. If you want to reach this muscle, try using a convex edge and a small tool to get in deep. You may need someone to do this area for your because it is so hard to reach but easy to find.

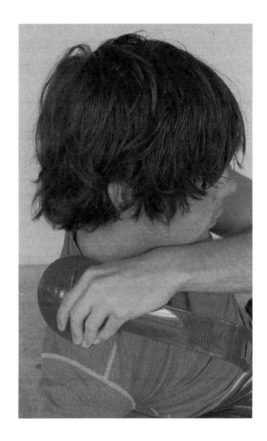

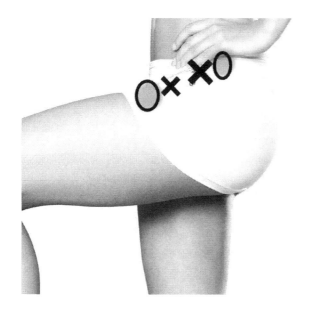
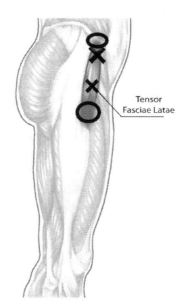

Tensor
Fasciae Latae

Tensor Fasciae Late

If you have knee or hip issues, this muscle needs to be treated. It is smaller than the other muscles nearby, but when dysfunctional, can send a lot of pain to nearby areas. It is connected to the IT Band so if it is dysfunctional, you will have instability from the hip, all the way down to the knee. The knee will be unstable and prone to degeneration.

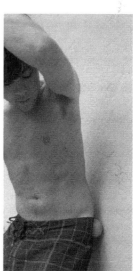

Trigger Point Treatment:

Lay on your side with your knees up and your knees bent. Put a lacrosse ball between the floor and this muscle and slowly roll it out.

Also, use a lacrosse ball against a wall.

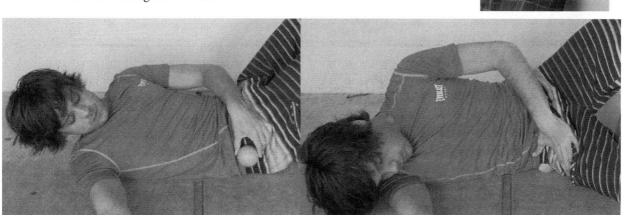

Scraping Treatment:

Stand straight with good pelvic posture (contract Abdominals and Glutes), then scrape this muscle out. Scrape over the whole muscle and try to find dysfunctional fascia. (The picture below depicts me not using lotion. You must remove your pants to scrape this muscle out. The picture below only shows where you need to scrape.)

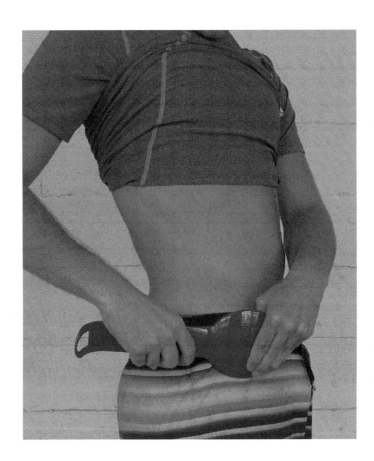

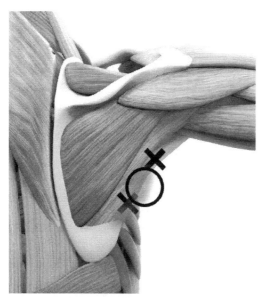
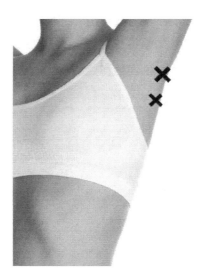

Teres Major

This muscle shares the same actions as the Latissimus Dorsi. It loves to develop painful knots in response to shoulder injuries.

Trigger Point Treatment:
Grab the wad of muscle behind the arm pit and feel for trigger points. You can also use a lacrosse ball against the floor to massage out this muscle at its insertion on the scapula (shoulder blade).

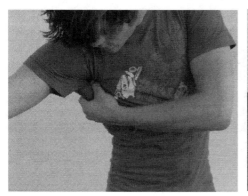
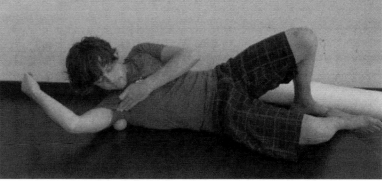

Scraping Treatment:
Lift up your arm to the side, and have someone scrape this muscle out. Stay on the "wing" portion that hangs under your arm pit; this is where the muscle lies. You can also scrape the area where the muscle attaches on the scapula. This area has a lot of muscles diverging in one spot, with various angles of pull acting on it, so it is a prime candidate for scar tissue build-up.

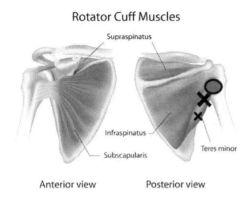

Rotator Cuff Muscles

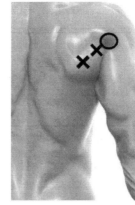

Teres Minor

This is a muscle that is overworked due to the fact that most of the shoulder muscles are internal rotators, and this little guy, along with the Infraspinatus, is primarily responsible for externally rotating the arm (they have a big job to do considering their size! This means that these two muscles are usually weak or inhibited, and full of trigger points.

Trigger Point Treatment:

Use a lacrosse ball against a wall. Keep your arm by your side and, after finding the Infraspinatus, go a little lower to massage this muscle on the outer border of the scapula. This muscle can have some pretty intense trigger points that can be very tender! Can be very sensitive, but well worth the pain.

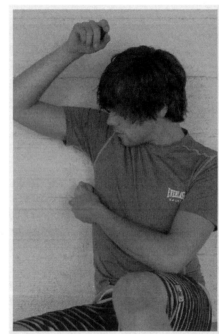
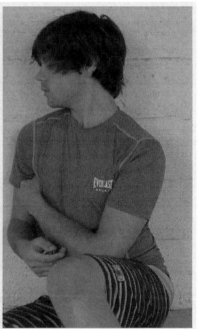

Scraping Treatment:

Have to have it done by someone else. Nearly impossible to scrape it yourself. Use a small convex tool work out the adhesions. Lay on a bed, on your stomach, on the edge of the bed with your arm hanging off the side. This is the best position to scrape this muscle.

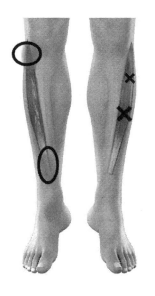
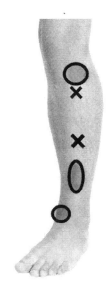

Tibialis Anterior

This is an important muscle with lots of responsibilities. This muscle is easily overworked because of its tough job. It not only brings the foot up towards the knee, but it also is a key mover in some ankle movements. This muscle needs to be healthy and functional in order to have good walking gait dynamics.

Trigger Point Treatment:
This muscle is easy to find because the muscle is easy to feel and easy to reach. Even though it is a thin muscle, it can have some deep trigger points that are hard to find.

The best ways to massage these trigger points out is to use a stainless steel water bottle filled with hot water. Roll this muscle slowly on the bottle and you will hit every single trigger point. Another option is to use a small foam roller.

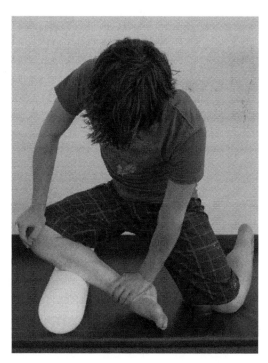

Scraping Treatment:

This muscle is very important muscle to scrape for most kinds of foot and ankle injuries. Watch out for the nerve that travels near the tendon of this muscle, near the ankle. Go soft and slow and stick to the areas in the pictures and you will be good to go. If you go softly at first, you will usually always find the nerves you need to avoid. If the pain you feel does not feel "needed" or "good pain", then do not do it. I always seem to find some kind of fascial dysfunction in this muscle and also the extensor tendon sheaths that its tendon passes under.

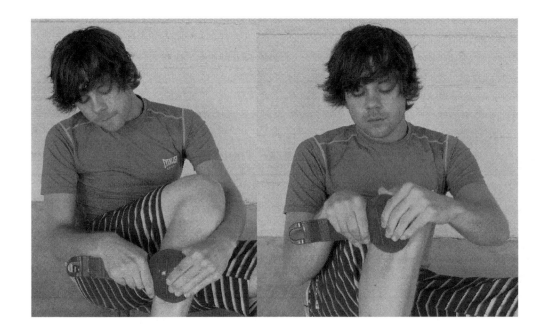

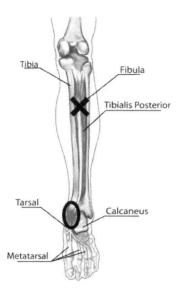

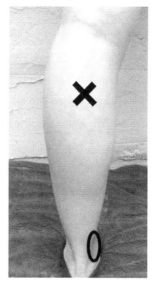

Tibialis Posterior

This deep calf muscle is responsible for ankle and foot movements. This muscle must be working properly if you want to have good walking gait mechanics. This muscle needs to be able to absorb the shock from the ground properly. If this muscle is not in good working order, you're at risk for degeneration of many structures that do not like to heal quickly. The problem with this muscle is that it is very deep.

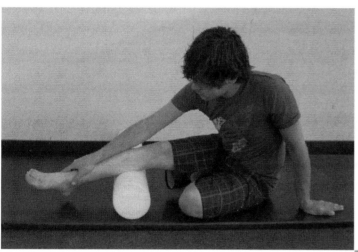

Trigger Point Treatment:
The only way to really reach this area is to use a rolling pin (or other comparable trigger point rolling stick). If you have blood clots or are at risk for them, do not try to work out the trigger points in this muscle.

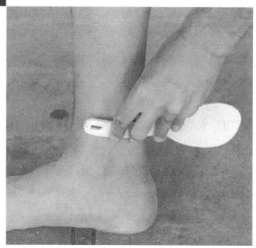

Scraping Treatment:
Working on the tendons of this muscle can cause some good relief. Also, the tendon sheath of this muscle can become sticky with scar tissue and instead of being fluid and lubricated, the tendon sheath becomes gritty and sticky. Work these areas out nice and slow with a small flat edge tool.

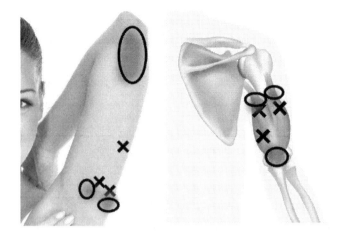

Triceps Brachii

This is an important muscle to treat for shoulder and elbow joint issues. It responds well to trigger point massage.

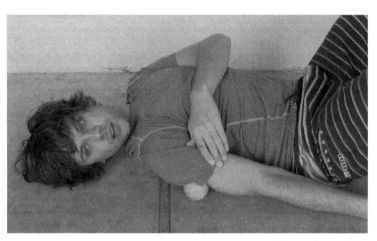

Trigger Point Treatment:
Use a lacrosse ball against a wall to massage out all of the trigger points. You can also lie down on the ground with the lacrosse ball to dig it into this muscle.

Scraping Treatment:
If you have a lot of pain in this area, or have tendonosis in this area, scrape the area entire muscle (and the tendon).

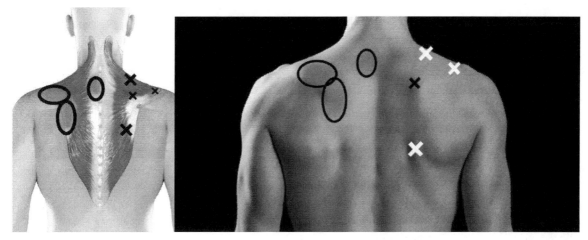

Trapezius

This muscle commonly feels good to massage. The reason is because it loves to become dysfunctional in the office worker. If you have to hunch over a desk all day, this muscle will be chronically lengthened and full of trigger points. Another implication to take into consideration is the fact that the Trapezius muscle deals with multiple angles of force. Some parts of the muscle make the scapula move one direction; others make the scapula move in the opposite direction. This can make the Trapezius's job extremely demanding and make it vulnerable to dysfunction. If the muscle is used frequently in someone with good posture and an active lifestyle, it is very hard for it to become dysfunctional. The instant you sit at a desk, and hunch over a keyboard, this muscle get put in a position that it should not be in. If this muscle has been bothering you for months on end and the trigger points do not seem to want to go away, try to release the Serratus Anterior and Pectoralis Minor. If that helps, also try doing shoulder rolls and shrugs every hour or so to get the muscle back into shape. Technically, it will not be technically "stronger", but more articulate with its movements (fine tuning your neurofacilitation mechanisms).

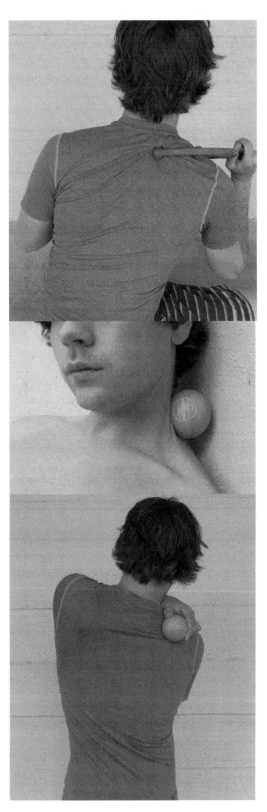

Trigger Point Treatment:
There are many trigger point treatment options. Use a Lacrosse ball against a wall. Also use a foam roller across the upper back. Back buddy stick can work as well for some of the big trigger points.

Scraping Treatment:
It works well to scrape this area. Do big broad strokes with a big straight edge tool over the whole muscle. Use a convex edge to work on some of the scar tissue build up areas.

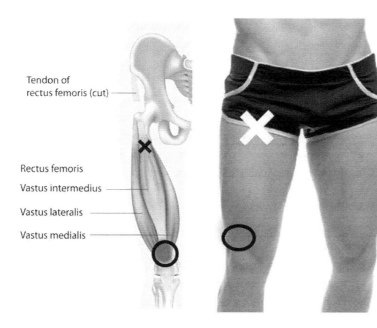

Vastus Intermedius

This muscle is very easy muscle to treat. It is right under the Rectus Femoris, on top of the thigh.

Tendon of rectus femoris (cut)

Rectus femoris
Vastus intermedius
Vastus lateralis
Vastus medialis

Trigger Point Treatment:

Use a rolling pin to roll out any trigger points. This muscle will be nearly impossible to massage if the Rectus Femoris has been dysfunctional for months. Just keep rolling this area out slowly. You can also use a foam roller, but rolling pin is better.

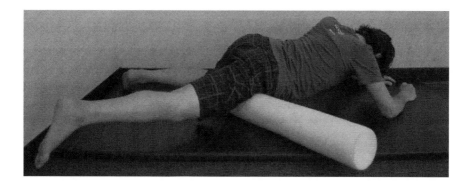

Scraping Treatment:

Not needed. Treat the Rectus Femoris scraping areas and you will be good to go.

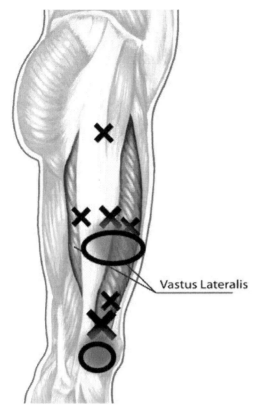

Vastus Lateralis

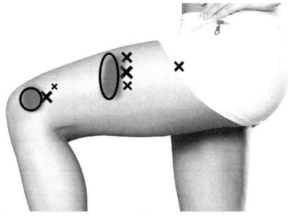

Vastus Lateralis

This muscle is a huge trouble maker! This muscle loves to be dysfunctional and even has trigger points in healthy individuals. If you have torn your meniscus or damaged any ligaments in the knee, you can almost always be sure that this muscle will be dysfunctional. It is big and strong.

It is responsible for sending pain down the outer edge of the leg, mimicking "IT Band Syndrome". Some argue that the trigger points in this muscle cause the pain experienced in IT Band Syndrome. When this muscle is shortened, it can cause the knee to "click" - it pulls the Patella against the lateral condyle of the Tibia, and when the patella hits this area, makes a noise from grinding against it. If you have patellae femoral syndrome, this muscle will be dysfunctional beyond belief.

Trigger Point Treatment:

Lots of treatment options. It can be hard to treat because the trigger points do not like to release as easily as other muscles. Use Rolling Pin, Lacrosse Ball, and Foam Roller. This muscle needs consistent treatment to see pain relief results from treating this muscle.

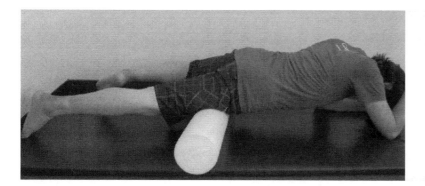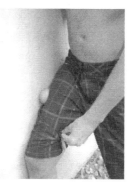

Scraping Treatment:

It is very important to treat this muscle with scraping. Scrape the whole muscle a couple of times and feel where the grainy texture is. You will find an area 1/3 the length of the thigh, near the knee. Also, scrape the whole attachment area and other areas noted in the pictures. This treatment can make you cry because it is very sensitive!

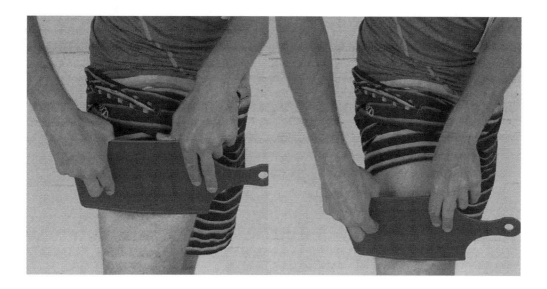

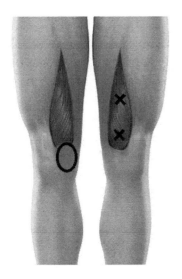
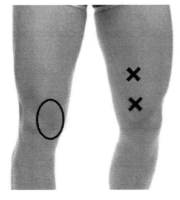

Vastus Medialis

This muscle is very important muscle for proper walking gait and knee stability. This muscle has the huge responsibility of pulling the patella (knee cap) medially while you walk. This can be stressful for the muscle if the opposing stabilizer, the Vastus Lateralis, is stronger (whether from more pronounced neuromuscular facilitation or from hypertrophy). What we want to do is fix the dysfunction and make it stronger. This muscle's exercises can be found in a later chapter called "Preventative Exercises".

Trigger Point Treatment:

I love hitting this muscle with a rolling pin or from a big foam roller. This muscle is never as dysfunctional as the Vastus Lateralis (which is usually a trouble-maker when it comes to knee pain). You will find the trigger points pretty quickly and be able to treat them pretty easily.

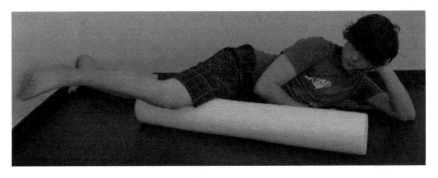

Scraping Treatment:

This is an easy area to scrape and helps quite a bit if you have Plicae Syndrome or MCL Tear. Simply use a big tool, either concave or straight edged, and scrapes the whole muscle. It is very easy to find and easy to treat.

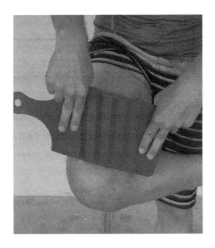

Third Step of MSTR: Kinetic Chain Stretches

In this section, we will learn how to elongate the fascia sheets to work out any dysfunctional kinks they may have developed over the course of your chronic inflammatory injury. This will fix your posture, release nerve entrapment, increase nutrient exchange to the muscles, and so much more. These stretches are very important if you want to have long-term relief from any injury.

It is very important to do these stretches after you have fixed the trigger points and worked out the cross-link fascia adhesions. If you were to do these kinetic chain stretches without working out the trigger points and cross-link fascia adhesions, you can make your injury much worse and cause further trigger point development.

In order to do these stretches safely, it is important to follow all the rules below so that you do not hurt yourself. These stretches can work miracles if done right, but can cause re-injury if done improperly.

Stretching Guidelines:

- Warm up. After a hot shower, swimming, or after bicycling is a great time to do these stretches. If you are in too much pain to exercise, try to do the stretches after a hot shower. Try to walk around, as much as your pain will allow, before doing the stretches. You need to warm up the fascia so that it will not contract, and instead relax. Having your tissues warmed up, either from lightly working out or from being in a warm environment, is the best way to prepare the tissues. Saunas are also a great option for warming up the fascia you will be stretching.

- Do the stretches later in the day. It is best to do them a few hours before bed.

- You only have to do your prescribed stretches (found in "Individual Injuries" chapter) once a day.

- Do not attempt to do the stretches if you have not followed the chronic pain diet as mentioned earlier in this book for at least two weeks.

- Do not attempt these stretches if you have not released the trigger points and cross-link adhesions. It is best to do the trigger point and cross-link adhesion work for two weeks (sometimes longer!) before attempting these stretches.

- If something feels like its "tearing", it probably is. If you feel burning pain or excessive pain of any kind, you are pushing the stretch too far and you probably did some damage.

Every stretch needs to be done nice and slowly. Do not jump into the stretches and try to stretch as hard and far as you can.

- After your pain is gone, try doing the stretches 2-3 times a week to keep the pain from coming back. After you are back to full health, you do not have to do the stretches anymore. But make sure your diet is perfect! Otherwise, the pain can return.

- If you have too much fruit or sugar, these stretches can be dangerous. People who have lots of sugar in their diet have dehydrated and inflamed fascia. Make sure you stick to the diet and drink plenty of water to make these stretches work.

- You should feel some discomfort from these stretches. They should not hurt, but they should not feel good. They should take some effort and you should feel a long stretch through the body.

- Do the stretches on both sides of the body. If your left foot hurts, do the stretches for all the kinetic chains involved in the foot for both your left and right foot. Even pain free areas far away from the injury can be causing your pain.

What these stretches do is stretch fascia, not so much muscle. However, if the muscles are not dysfunctional, they will benefit from these stretches.

Throughout the body there are chains of muscles that are all connected with fascia. Remember that fascia is a connective tissue that forms the framework of your body. These chains of muscles are kinetic chains. The strength and functionality of a kinetic chain depends on functionality of the entire chain. If one part of the chain is "kinked" or "contracted", the whole kinetic chain suffers. This is how pain can spread to other areas.

A kinetic chain can confuse people sometimes, because how in the world are individual/separate muscles connected in a so called "chain"? It is because the fascia is continuous, from deep inside the muscle, all the way to the bone it attaches to. The fascia can go right through bone, and connect to a muscle on the other side. It can also wrap around a bone. For example, in the heel bone, the calf muscle's tendon goes through the heel bone, and out the bottom of the foot, which becomes the plantar fascia. Fascia is continuous and connects literally everything together. If fascia was not connecting separate muscle together, our bodies would be extremely weak; this is why it is so crucial to have it functioning properly.

In order to stretch the fascia in a kinetic chain, we must elongate every muscle in the chain but remain within its healthy range of motion. Unlike conventional stretching, fascia stretching does not put the muscle in an unhealthy or forced "stretch", so that instead of stretching muscle, we will stretch the fascia between and around the muscle. This is where the dysfunction is after we take care of the trigger points and the cross-link adhesions. The fascia needs to be held in this elongated position for at least a minute so that it responds favorably. Fascia is similar to taffy, and when you slowly elongate it, it likes to stay that way. If there are any postural issues, these stretches will be great as a diagnostic tool to see where the postural problem has originated from.

Some stretches will feel good and natural and you will not feel much of a stretch. This means that that the kinetic chain is healthy. You do not have to do these stretches if they feel this way. If you have pain anywhere, you will have quite a few kinetic chains that need to be stretched, so do not get too excited just yet. There is a lot of work to come!

Sometimes a kinetic chain will feel good on one side of the body, but the opposite side of the body (left vs. right) will have dysfunction. Be sure to focus on the dysfunctional kinetic chains (ones that feel uncomfortable to stretch) until both sides of the body feel the same amount of stretch.

Every injury will have different areas of dysfunction depending on the person. I will give you a list of kinetic chain stretches to work on in the "Individual Injuries" chapter, and it is your job to go through all the stretches daily for about 2 weeks. After that much time, you will know where the extremely dysfunctional kinetic chains are located. Work on these until they are functional. At most you should only have to do these stretches for 6-8 weeks. Some people only need them for 2 weeks for small injuries. If your injury has been around for years, you may need to do these stretches for a long time.

Feel around for trigger point development in the muscles in the days after starting to do these stretches. If tender points develop out of nowhere, you need to take a step back and stop the stretches, and go back to the trigger point. When they are completely taken care of, and not tender, try the stretches again.

Spinal Kinetic Stretches

The first six stretches of the Kinetic Chain Stretches will be concerned with bringing function to the chains associated closest to the spine. These stretches are very important due to there close relation to the "core" of the body. If there is any dysfunction in the fascia that surrounds the spine (or muscles of the spine) then you are going to have problems.

These stretches are better done after lunch time due to the fact that the spine is more warmed up and malleable after this time. Do not try to do these stretches in the morning.

In order to get proper results from these stretches, and other kinetic chain stretches, you will have to learn a special technique. It has to do with making a double chin, without moving the head forward or bending the neck. What this does is align your neck and muscle of the neck so that the fascia can be manipulated properly.

Look at the pictures below to get an idea of what this technique looks like:

Good Posture

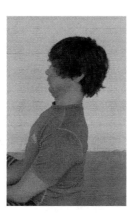

Bad Posture

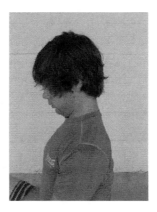

Stretch One

Upper Neck

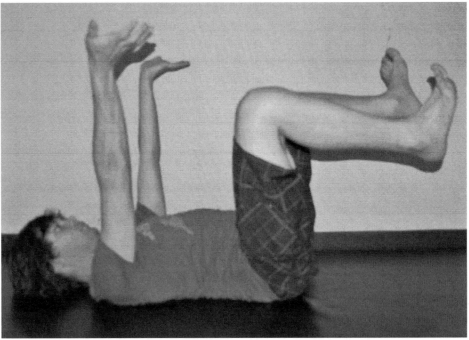

- Go on your back and assume position in the picture above.

- Lift head slightly off the ground, make a double chin, but do not bend your neck. You want your spine to be straight and this is only done by making a double chin without bending your neck. And when you lift your head off the ground, it should be less than an inch, not much.

- Push your hands forward with your arms stretched out as hard as you can (literally push your arms forward, without movement).

- Then bend your fingers back and lock your elbows until they are straight.

- Tighten up your abdominal muscles and squeeze your bottom (pinch a penny, so to speak).

- Evert the feet (make the bottom of the feet go outward).

- Keep the back flat against the ground.

- Keep the knees at 90 degree angles. The thighs should be perpendicular to the floor, and the lower leg should be parallel with the ground.

- With practice this stretch will become easy (it can be hard to hit all the points above on your first try).

- Hold the stretch for 30 seconds, rest for 10 seconds, then hold for another 30 seconds.

Stretch Two

Lower Neck

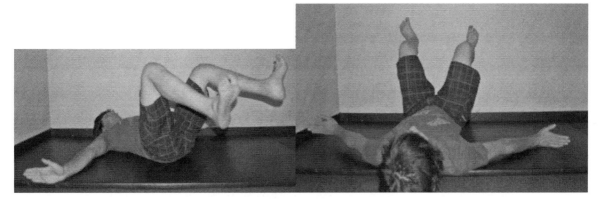

- Go on your back and assume position in the picture above.

- Lift head slightly off the ground, make a double chin, but do not bend your neck. You want your spine to be straight and this is only done by making a double chin without bending your neck. And when you lift your head off the ground, it should be less than an inch, not much.

- Push your hands downward with your arms stretched out at 45 degree angles on the sides of your body, and push down as hard as you can (literally push your arms downward, without movement. It is a static force. If you push down with your arms, you will contract certain muscles that will cause a release in the neck musculature).

- Then bend your fingers back and lock your elbows until they are straight. Point your inner elbow (the arm pit of the elbow, so to speak) up towards the sky.

- Tighten up your abdominal muscles and squeeze your bottom (pinch a penny, so to speak).

- Evert the feet (make the bottom of the feet go outward).

- Keep the back flat against the ground.

- Keep the knees at 90 degree angles, the thighs should be perpendicular to the floor, and the lower leg should be parallel with the ground.

- With practice this stretch will become easy (it can be hard to hit all the points above on your first try).

- Hold the stretch for 30 seconds, rest for 10 seconds, then hold for another 30 seconds.

Stretch Three

Middle Thoracic

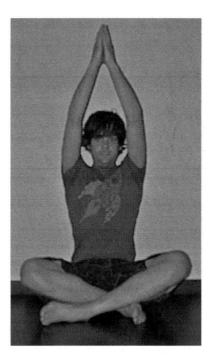

- Assume the position in the picture above.

- Make your spine straight and in line with your arms. It helps to look at your profile with a mirror. Make sure that your back is as straight as possible.

- Push your hands up towards the sky, and also press your hands together as hard as possible.

- Raise your chest upward.

- Make a double chin without bending the neck downward.

- Push upward with a lot of effort!

- Hold for 30 seconds, rest for 10, and then hold for another 30 seconds.

Stretch Four

Lower Thoracic

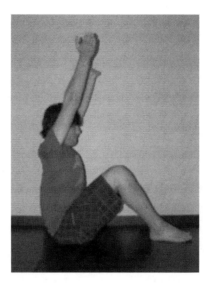

- Assume the position in the picture above.

- Contract your glues and abdominals so that your pelvis is in its proper position. This will put your spine in an ideal position for this stretch.

- Make sure your knees are at 90 degree angles and close to one another.

- Make a double chin without bending the neck downward.

- Extend your fingers and wrist out as far as you can to your sides (as seen in the picture).

- Extend your elbows until they are straight and causing your arms to point straight up to the sky.

- Then, push upward with your arms. Use as much force as you can to push against absolutely nothing. This is a static force, so do not try to go beyond your natural range of motion, just try to hold the position forcefully, as if you are about to catch a rock from falling on your head.

- It is very easy to put your legs too close or too far away from your body which causes your pelvis to be out of alignment, which would cause a bad stretch. Be sure to assume the position in the picture to the best of your ability, and keep those glutes contracted so that the pelvis is in a good position.

- Hold for 30 seconds, then rest for 10, then hold for another 30 seconds.

Stretch Five

Upper Lumbar

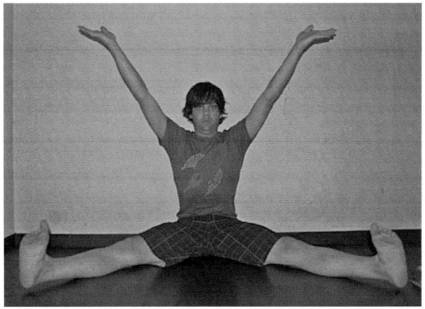

- Assume the position in the picture above.

- Invert the feet (position the bottom of the foot towards your midline).

- Lock the knees so that the knee joint is straight. You can contract your quadriceps to accomplish this.

- Push your pelvis forward slightly. Do this by leaning your whole body forward. When you are in this position it is easy to lean backward. Keep away from this and try to make your spine perpendicular to the ground.

- Bring the chest up a little.

- Keep the arms up and out, extend the fingers and extend the elbows.

- Push upward. Imagine trying to catch a huge rock that is about to fall on your head.

- Hold the stretch for 30 seconds, rest for 10, then hold for 30 seconds again.

Stretch Six

Lower Lumbar

Do not do this stretch if your lower back pain is severe or if you have active sciatica! Let it subside then try this stretch out again.

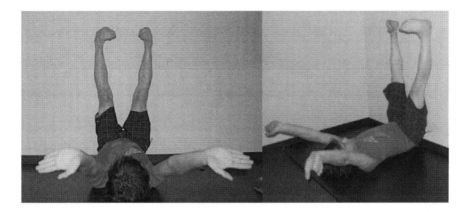

- Assume the position in the picture above. Lie down on the floor next to a wall, then swing your legs up against the wall.

- Lift head slightly off the ground, make a double chin, but do not bend your neck. You want your spine to be straight and this is only done by making a double without bending your neck. And when you lift your head off the ground, it should be less than an inch, not much.

- Push your legs down into your pelvis. You need to imagine your legs sinking into your pelvis. Let gravity push them slowly into position while you are against the wall.

- Invert the feet (point the bottom of the feet towards your midline).

- Lock the knees by contracting the Quadriceps muscles. Also, while inverting your feet, try to bring them towards your knee.

- Internally rotate your legs. Do this by trying to point your knees forward or towards each other. Or by pointing your feet at each other (this should be a subtle rotation, not very extreme, look at the pictures and notice how my feet are pointing at each other slightly).

- Tighten your abdominals so that your back is flat against the ground.

- Push your arms above your head with your fingers extended and your elbows locked and straight.

- Hold for 30 seconds, relax for 10, and then hold for 30 more seconds. Do not forget to breath!! Do not hold your breath while doing this stretch.

Kinetic Chain Stretches for the rest of the body

In the following pages you will find the rest of the kinetic chain stretches that are for areas besides the spine.

Stretch Seven

Scalene Stretch

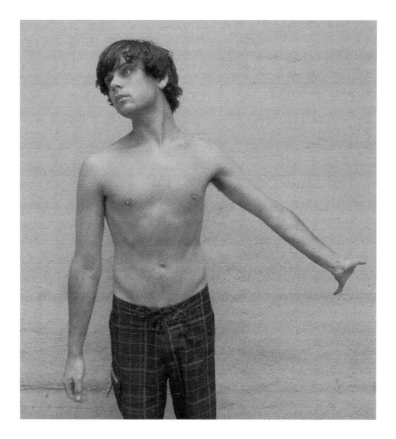

- Rotate head away from the side being stretched.

- Tilt head ever so slightly away from the side being stretched.

- Puff your chest out a little bit.

- Extend arm out 45 degrees to the side of your body.

- Extend the fingers back as far as you can.

- Extend the elbow joint as far as possible.

- At this point you can do the final step, drop the shoulder. Dropping the shoulder will complete the stretch, and you should feel it from the tips of your fingers all the way up to your neck.

- Hold for 10 seconds, then rest for 10 seconds, then hold it again for 30 seconds.

Stretch Eight

Internal Rotator Stretch

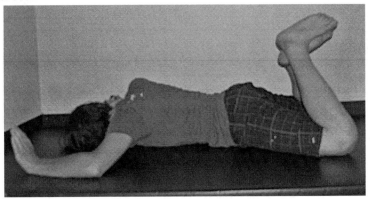

I tore both Labrums on my shoulder, so most will be able to get their shoulder closer to the ground than I can in the photo.

- Assume position in the picture above.

- Make sure head is facing away from the side being stretched.

- Extend fingers upward.

- Spread knees slight away from each other and press your feet together.

- Contract the Glutes.

- Use the arm on the side not being stretched to lift that side of your body up, and push the side being stretched, shoulder and chest, down into the ground.

- You want to imagine that you need to lift the wrist with the fingers extended off the ground. This will cause the external rotators in your shoulder to contract, thereby releasing the internal rotators. It should be a subtle contraction though. Try to lift your arm up without moving it.

- Go deeper into the stretch by pushing your shoulder deeper into the ground, or lifting up the other side of the body that is not being stretched.

- Hold for 10 seconds, relax for 10, and then hold it for 30 seconds.

Stretch Nine

External Rotator Stretch

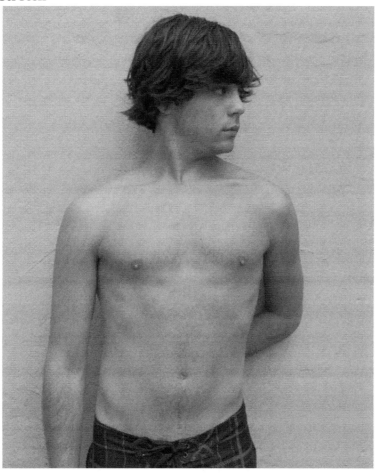

- Stand with back against a wall.

- Put arm completely behind your back slowly; with your palm facing the wall If you have rotator cuff issues, be sure to have completely taken care of all the trigger points in the Infraspinatus and teres minor before doing this stretch. And do the stretch slowly and carefully.

- Turn your head towards the side being stretched. Make a slight double chin for proper neck position.

- Drop your shoulder slightly. If this causes pain, go only as far as you can go such as in my picture above. If you can, try to drop your shoulder as far down as you comfortably can go.

- Now you will press your palm into the wall. This will contract your internal rotator muscles thereby relaxing the external rotator muscles.

- Hold for 10 seconds, rest for 10 seconds, and then hold it again for 30 seconds.

Stretch Ten

Upper Neck Extender Stretch

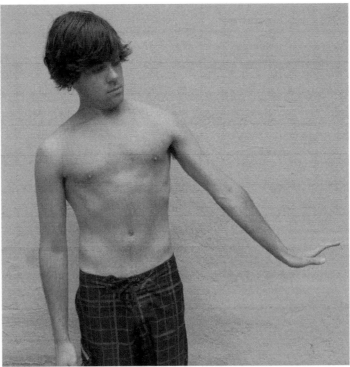

- Tilt head away from side being stretched.

- Rotate head toward the side being stretched.

- Extend the fingers as far back as possible.

- Extend elbow joint as far as possible.

- Raise arm out to side at 45 degree angle.

- Now you will complete the stretch with dropping the shoulder on the side being stretched. You will feel the stretch from the back of your head, all the way down to the tips of the fingers.

- Hold for 10 seconds, rest for 10 seconds, and then hold it again for 30 seconds.

Stretch Eleven

Mid Back Stretch

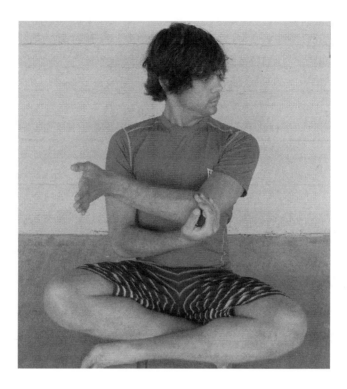

- Assume position in the picture.

- Raise chest up.

- Reach arm across chest with elbow bent and fingers extended backwards.

- Turn head towards arm being stretched while keeping a slight double chin and proper neck posture.

- Drop the shoulder down while pushing the shoulder forward.

- Hold stretch for 10 seconds, rest for 10 seconds, and then hold it again for 30 seconds.

Stretch Twelve

Lateral Back Stretch

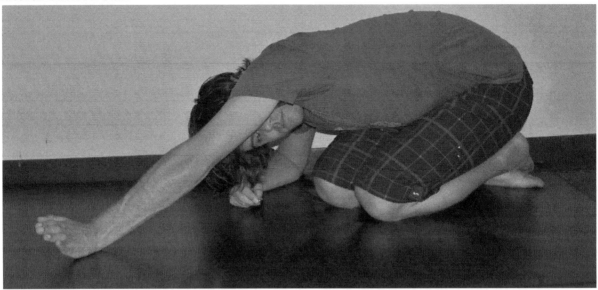

This stretches the kinetic chain that is home to the Latissimus Dorsi and Oblique muscles. Make sure your knees are on some kind of a mat or padding, and not a hard wood floor.

- Assume the position in the picture above.

- Turn your head towards the side being stretched. Do not tilt or bend the neck, you must rotate it towards the side being stretched.

- Extend fingers and lock the elbow. Also, externally rotate the arm by pointing your hand outward, as seen in the photo.

- Hunch your back slowly until you feel a stretch from your fingers to your lower back.

- Now, contract the oblique muscles on the opposite side (the side not being stretched). This will cause your spine to bend laterally (to the side) so that the side being stretched becomes more lengthened.

- Now push up with your arm above your head. Try to push the palm away from your body as well, as hard as you can (but build up pressure slowly).

- Now hold this stretch for 10 seconds, rest for 10 seconds, and then hold again for 30 seconds.

Stretch Thirteen

Pectoral and Front of Shoulder Stretch

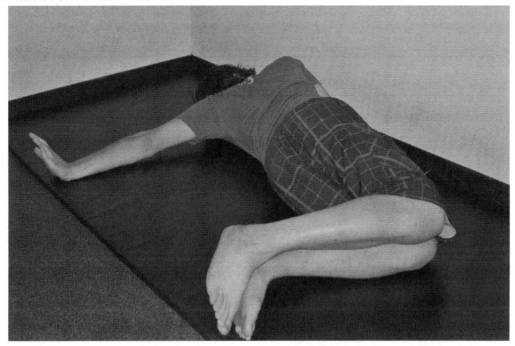

- Assume the position in the picture above. My shoulders have torn labrums so understand that you will be able to push your shoulder into the ground. Some people that have frozen shoulder/chronic rotator cuff problems/torn labrums will only be able to drop the shoulder into the ground as far as seen in the picture.

- Turn your head towards the side not being stretched.

- Extend fingers upward towards the sky and extend the elbow.

- Contract your glutes by "pinching a penny".

- Make sure that your legs are in the same position mine are in. This will twist your body so the stretch is easier to do.

- Use the arm that is on the side not being stretched to lift up that side of the body. You will need to do this in order to press your shoulder into the ground (on the side being stretched). Go into this portion of the stretch very slowly and be careful.

- Extend the arm outward and up towards the sky subtly. You want to contract the back muscles a bit so that the pectoral muscles will release.

- Hold the stretch for 10 seconds, rest for 10 seconds, and then hold for 30 seconds.

Stretch Fourteen

Elbow Flexor Stretch

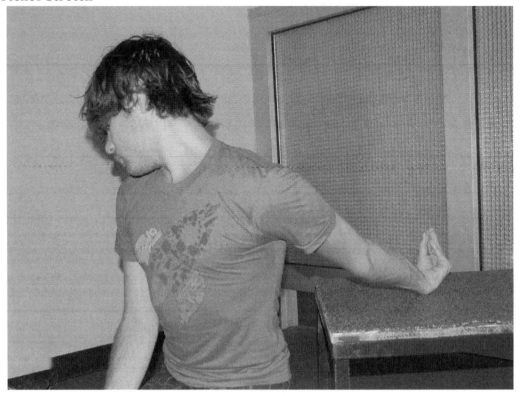

- Assume the position in the picture above and put your arm on a table while sitting in a chair, or find a stool and place it next to your ground so you can do the position as seen in the picture.

- Turn your head and tilt it away from the side being stretched.

- Drop the shoulder.

- Extend the elbow.

- Put your hand in the position as seen in the picture. It is a "full hand pinch" and also flex the wrist so that the hand is pointing to the sky.

- Now what you want to do is focus on extending the elbow and dropping the shoulder. This will release your elbow flexors.

- Hold the stretch for 10 seconds, rest for 10 seconds, and then hold for 30 more seconds.

Stretch Fifteen

Elbow Extender Stretch

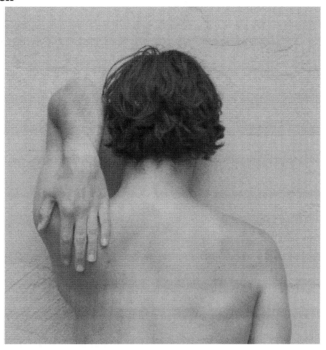

- Face a wall and bring your arm up and over your head. Assume the position in the photograph above but with your elbow touching the wall.

- Lean your weight slowly against the wall, letting the Tricep muscle slowly go into a nice stretch.

- Now, flex your elbow joint by flexing your Bicep muscles so that the Tricep will release.

- Hold for 10 seconds, rest for 10 seconds, and then hold it again for 30 seconds.

Stretch Sixteen

Wrist and Forearm Stretches

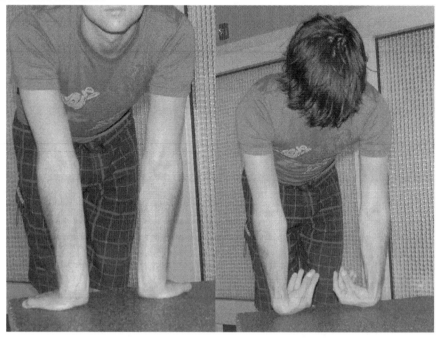

- Find a table or stool or empty area of ground that you can use to assume the two positions as seen in the pictures above

- Extend the elbows as far as possible

- If you are doing the stretch as seen in the picture on the left, try to extend the back of your hand and fingers up towards the sky. This will release the wrist flexors

- If you are doing the stretch as seen in the picture on the right, try to flex the fingers up towards the sky, and flex the wrists as seen in the picture. This will release the wrist extensors

- Hold each stretch for 10 seconds, then rest for 10 seconds, then hold the stretch again for 30 seconds

Stretch Seventeen

Hip Flexor Stretch

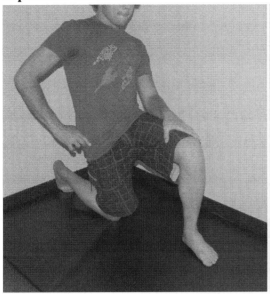 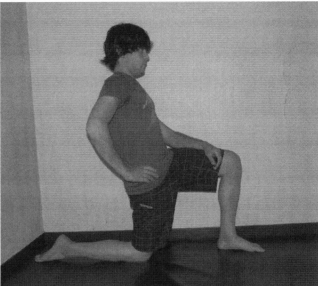

- Assume the position in the picture above

- Make sure that you have a piece of soft padding or foam under your knee. Pillows work for this purpose

- Make a slight double chin and keep your chest up and back straight

- Now the important part: Contract the abdominals and glutes so that the hip flexors will release and stretch

- Bend your torso away from the leg that is behind you. Tilt your spine laterally away from the side being stretched. The hip flexors attach to the spine, so this is very crucial

- If possible, try to find a wall or stationary object to put against the inner edge of the foot that is behind you. This will inhibit rotation of the hip that is unfavorable when trying to stretch the hip flexors

- Hold the stretch for 20 seconds, relax for 10, then hold for another 30 seconds

Stretch Eighteen

Knee Extender Stretch

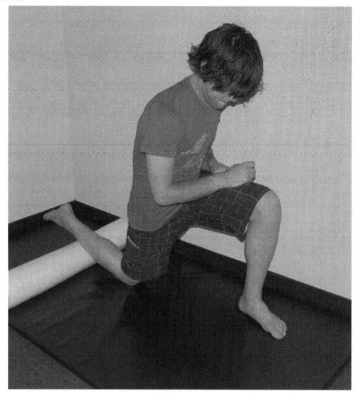

- Assume position in the picture above. Use a piece of padding or pillow under your knee. Then find a second piece of padding or object to place under your foot. In the picture above I am using a foam roller.

- Unlike the hip flexor stretch, we do not want to flex the abdominals and glutes. Instead we want to extend the hip just enough to cause a stretch in the knee extensors

- Lift your foot up towards the sky with static strength. You do not need to move the foot, but you need to "try" to lift it up. This will engage the hamstring muscles and will cause a release in the knee extenders.

- Hold the stretch for 20 seconds, rest for 10 seconds, and then hold it again for 30 seconds.

Stretch Nineteen

Hip Extender Stretch

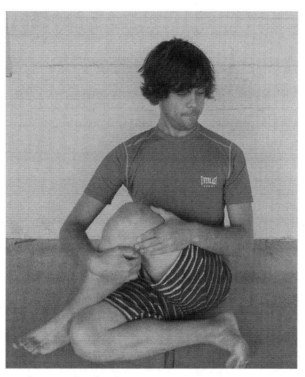

- Assume position in the picture above.

- Keep chest up and head position neutral. Make a slight double chin.

- Use the force of your muscles to bring your knee towards your chest. Then use your hands to hold the knee in the position. Keep muscle tension active by bring your knee up towards your chest. This will release the Hip Extender Muscles.

- Hold for 20 seconds, rest for 10 seconds, and then hold it again for 30 seconds.

Stretch Twenty

Hamstring Stretches

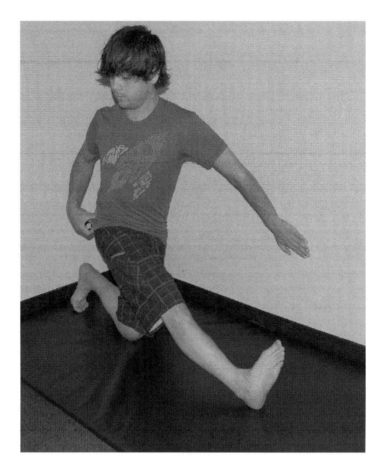

Outer Hamstring Stretch:

- Assume position in picture.

- Invert foot (point the bottom of the foot towards the opposite leg).

- Bring Foot back while inverting it. Do not try to stretch the calf; you should feel only a small stretch in the calf while doing this.

- Next, contract the Quadriceps muscles in order to straighten and extend the Knee joint.

- Lift up your chest and then slowly lower your stomach and torso down to the leg being stretched. Also, slowly rotate the chest towards the leg being stretched. Slowly bring your chest further down to the leg while contracting the quadriceps so that the Hamstring muscles will release.

- Hold this stretch for 20 seconds, then rest for 10 seconds, then stretch again for 30 seconds.

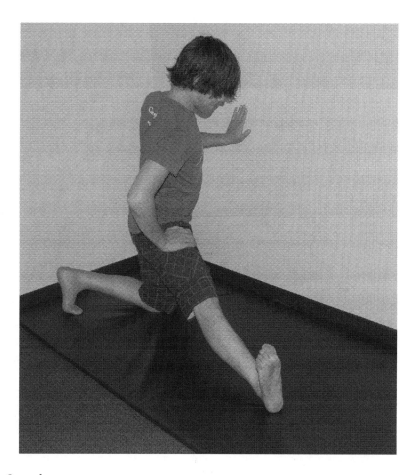

Inner Hamstring Stretch:

- Assume position in picture.

- Evert foot (point the bottom of the foot away from the midline of the body; outward).

- Bring Foot back while Everting it. Do not try to stretch the calf; you should feel only a small stretch in the calf while doing this.

- Next, contract the Quadriceps muscles in order to straighten and extend the Knee joint.

- Lift up your chest and then slowly lower your stomach and torso down to the leg being stretched. Also, slowly rotate the chest away from the leg being stretched.

- Slowly bring your stomach further down to the leg while contracting the quadriceps so that the Hamstring muscles will release.

- Hold this stretch for 20 seconds, then rest for 10 seconds, then stretch again for 30 seconds.

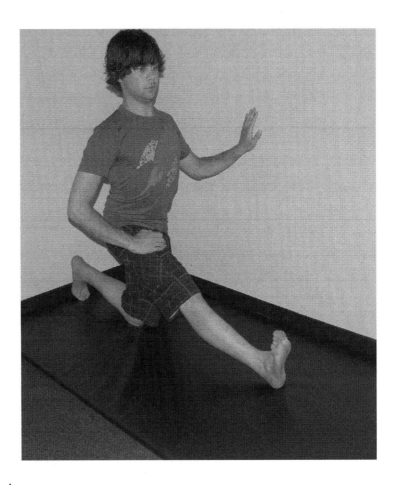

Middle Hamstring Stretch:

- Assume position in picture.

- Bring Foot back. Do not try to stretch the calf; you should feel only a small stretch in the calf while doing this.

- Next, contract the Quadriceps muscles in order to straighten and extend the Knee joint.

- Lift up your chest and then slowly lower your stomach and torso down to the leg being stretched.

- Slowly bring your chest further down to the leg while contracting the quadriceps so that the Hamstring muscles will release.

- Hold this stretch for 20 seconds, then rest for 10 seconds, then stretch again for 30 seconds.

Stretch Twenty One

Hip Rotator Stretch

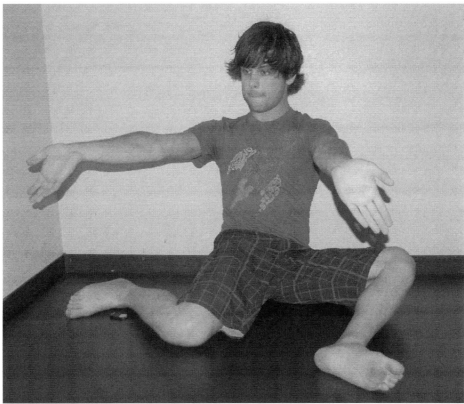

- Assume position slowly. If you have knee issues, be careful with this stretch or avoid it until the knee issues are all healed up.

- Focus on pushing the palms out and away from you.

- Make a slight double chin.

- Contract the Abdominals and Glutes in order to put your pelvis in a proper position. Then bring your rib cage down until you have proper posture.

- Next you need to tilt your chest and body towards the right leg. You also want to rotate slightly towards this leg as well.

- Now you will want to push your right buttock (leg that you are facing toward), down into the ground. This will rotate the femur more so and put the hip rotators in a deep stretch.

- Go very slowly! Hold this stretch for 20 seconds, then relax for 10, then hold the stretch again for 30 more seconds.

Stretch Twenty Two

Hip Adductor Stretches

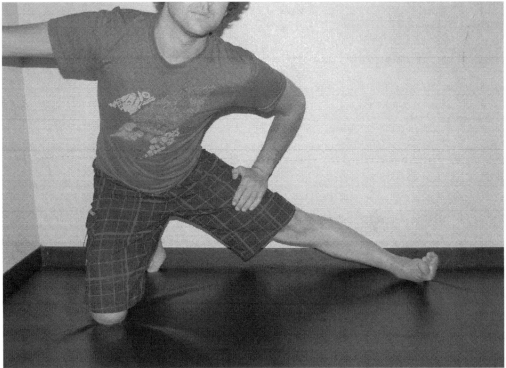

- Assume position in picture above

- Try to Evert the foot (keep the bottom faced away from the midline of the body, outward).

- Bring toes back.

- Extend Knee Joint.

- Contract the Hip Abductors. This is by "trying" to raise the leg from the ground, just without moving it. We need to contract those muscles a little so that the Hip Adductors can release.

- Hold this position for 10 seconds, then relax for 10 seconds, then hold it again for 30 seconds.

Stretch Twenty Three

Lower Leg Flexor Stretch

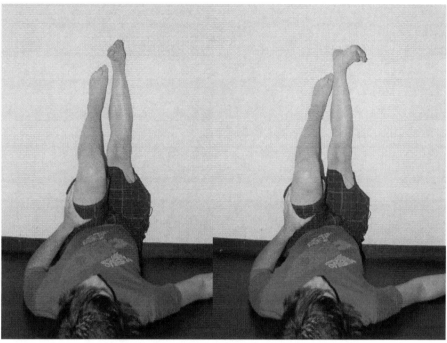

- Lie down next to a wall and kick your feet up against the wall.

- Push your butt into the wall slowly.

- Flatten your back by contracting your abs.

- Extend the knee joint on the side being stretched. This is done by contracting the quadriceps.

- Bring the toes and foot back towards your face.

- While doing this stretch, there are two variations. One is inverted, the other is everted. Inverted means that the foot bottom is facing towards the opposite leg. Everted means that the bottom of the foot is facing away from the midline of the body.

- Invert the foot while doing this stretch for 20 seconds (Picture on the left shows how to Invert the foot). Then Evert the foot while doing this stretch for 20 seconds (Picture on right shows how to Evert the foot). Rest for 20 seconds. Then choose whichever stretch was harder (Inverted or Everted) and stretch that position for another 20 seconds.

Stretch Twenty Four

Lower Leg Extensor Stretch

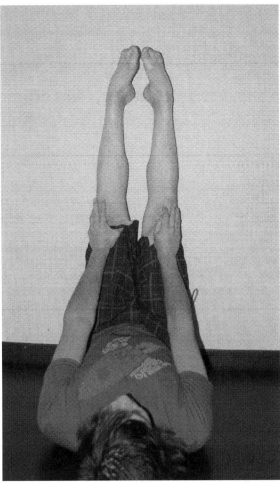

- Lie down next to a wall and kick your feet up against the wall.

- Extend Knee joints as far as possible.

- Point toes. You should feel a deep stretch in the anterior compartment of the lower leg (shin area).

- Hold the stretch for 20 seconds, then rest for 10 seconds, then hold again for 30 seconds.

Stretch Twenty Five

Deep Foot Flexor Stretch

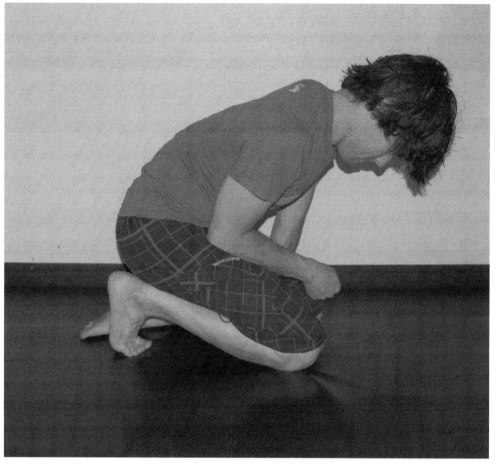

- Go Slowly!

- Get into the position in the picture above and slowly push into the stretch.

- Try to imagine your toes lifting up towards your knee (this will contract the toe extensors, thereby releasing the toe flexors.

- If you have severe plantar fasciitis or other issues, you need to be very careful with this stretch. It can cause a lot of damage if you have had a recent injury, but if not, it could fix a lot of pain issues. Just go very slowly.

- Hold the stretch for 20 seconds, rest for 10 seconds, and then hold it again for 30 seconds.

Individual Injuries

This chapter shows you a list of common injuries for each area of the body and how to fix them. The type of injury you have does not change the treatment too much. You will be diagnosing and treating each muscle in the area regardless, and you will find that some structures are more dysfunctional than others.

Whether you have front of shoulder pain or back of shoulder pain, you will still look at the same muscles. The reason why is because all the muscles work with each other. When one area is injured, all the structures like to become dysfunctional to "splint" the joints around the injury.

Someone with Achilles tendonitis and someone with chronic shin splints are going to have the same list of muscles to treat. This does not mean that they will be fixed in the same way. Once you start feeling the muscles, it will become apparent which ones need to be treated more than others. If half of the muscles on the list are extremely tender, work on those.

After you fix a dysfunctional muscle, you may have sporadic pains in other areas. This is because the body has already adapted to compensating for the dysfunctional structures. When you make a structure functional again, everything that is connected to the structure needs to adapt to its newly-fixed structures' functionality.

For instance, if you have chronic shoulder pain, such as a torn labrum, your subscapularis muscle is more than likely shortened, painful and extremely dysfunctional. After a couple sessions of therapy to the subscapularis, you may notice that you do not have the pain you're used to (and it has lessened!), but it has spread to a new area. Keep on going down the list of muscles for each injury and try to seek out more areas of dysfunction. After a while all of the pain patterns will change and the pain will hopefully diminish. Just hang in there and do not get discouraged. Your pain is there for a reason, and we need to fix what's causing it.

Keep feeling around for these new areas and treat them as they come. When all the areas are functional, your injury should be out of the downward spiral of chronic pain and should start to improve quickly (if not already).

If the therapies do not work, go to a professional to see what they can do. Just because you're scraping skills do not invoke substantial pain relief does not mean that it cannot help you. Go to a trained Graston ® therapist and see what results they can give you. If you do not have pain relief results, it is because you are looking the wrong area, you are not pressing hard enough (with trigger point massage), or because you have an underlying disorder/disease that is causing your results to be hindered. Be sure to check with a doctor before trying these therapies to be sure that they are safe to do with your current health and activity levels.

With every injury area, you will have a list of muscles to treat. This means go back to the "muscle guide" and figure out which muscles are more than likely dysfunctional for your pain. Next, treat all the trigger points in the muscles of the list. Start at the top of the list because the most commonly troublesome muscles will be first in the list.

After you have fixed the trigger points, try scraping the areas that were most dysfunctional. You do not need to scrape a whole lot, and it should take a lot less time than the trigger point therapy. Scraping is a very direct and aggressive form of therapy that does not have to be done in the same area every day. It should be done daily, but in differing areas.

Do scraping therapy once a day, but make sure that every day you will try to scrape a new muscle or area. You will find the trouble spots pretty quickly once you start feeling around with a scraping tool. Once you have tried scraping all the muscles for your individual injury over the course of about a week, you will know where the "big problem causing" areas are. Scrape these areas every day or every other day. It really depends on the area needing to be scraped. In some areas, such as the bottom of the foot, you can scrape twice a day at most. In some areas, you can only scrape once every three days! So try to mix it up and do not over do it if anything hurts. If it does, give it a break and come back to it in a few days.

Once you find out which muscles are dysfunctional, treat those daily. If only 5 muscles out of 15 are dysfunctional, just work on those for a while. After they are functional, over a week or two, check out the other muscles. You may find some dysfunction that you over looked before, or dysfunction that was created from compensation patterns. When you fix one area, all the areas around it have to be "reprogrammed" to work properly again, and this can cause some issues. So every week or so, check all the muscles under your "muscle list" for your "individual injury" so you can figure out if anything has gone awry.

If you get tons of pain relief for the first couple of weeks, then none after, you are not looking the right areas (or your diet is not consistently good). You need to go over the list of muscles and feel each one with your hands or a scraping tool and find out where the dysfunction lies.

When you have less pain and have been chasing after dysfunctional muscles for 2-3 weeks, you are now ready to do the kinetic chain stretches. Be sure to go back to the chapters and re-read the section on how to do kinetic chain stretches. Do all the stretches as outlined for your individual injury. As with the muscles and fascia adhesion treatments, kinetic chain stretches are a treatment and a diagnostic tool. You will soon notice that some stretches are more needed than other stretches. You will find that some stretches feel "good" or "needed". Continue with these kinetic chain stretches until the problem is completely gone.

If you re-injure an area, but you were already at the kinetic chain stretching stage, you will have to take a step back. You will need to give the area a couple days to a couple weeks of rest. Try doing trigger point work to the muscles again and slowly build up through all the steps of MSTR therapy. Re-injury can be extremely frustrating. Do not test your injury out of desperation. Start from square one and slowly begin treatment once again.

The Importance of Getting a Proper Diagnosis from a Professional

You cannot watch health TV shows or go online to get a diagnosis. Not for these kinds of injuries. You need to go to a health care professional and figure out what is wrong. There are so many methods that doctor's use, that is hands on, to figure out what is wrong with you. You cannot do these things over the phone or over the internet. See a real doctor in person.

You also need to rule out other disorders. Sometimes back pain is not just back pain, and could be signs of kidney dysfunction. You need to see a doctor to make sure that that pain you have is not something major.

This book is great at fixing chronic injuries that doctors have problems fixing. The types of problems that the doctor says "apply ice and it should go away in a month or so".... But then the pain is still there two years from now and driving you completely crazy. And the doctor cannot find anything else to blame for your pain. That's when you should use this book.

If you break your leg, go to a doctor. If your pain came out of nowhere, go to a doctor. Get it checked out first, and then use this book to fix it if the doctor can't.

Neck Pain

Muscles to Treat (biggest troublemakers first):

1. Sternocleidomastoid
2. Levator Scapulae
3. Splenius Capitis/Splenius Cervicis/Semispinalis Capitis
4. Trapezius (upper fibers)
5. Occipitalis
6. Scalene Group
7. Back Erectors

Kinetic Chain Stretches Needed:

1. Stretch 1
2. Stretch 2
3. Stretch 3
4. Stretch 4
5. Stretch 7
6. Stretch 10
7. Stretch 13
8. Stretch 14
9. Stretch 17
10. Stretch 20

Common Injuries to this Area:

Whiplash (pain after the injury has healed), Chronic Pain and Stiffness and Tightness, Levator Scapulae Strain, Cervical Disk Bulge

Effective Alternative Therapies:

Most Chronic Neck Pain: Active Release Technique ® (great for nerve entrapment in this area), Cross Friction Massage if area is localized in one point, Cold Laser Therapy ®, Chiropractic

Cervical Disk Bulge: Myofascial Release ®, Active Release Technique ®, Chiropractic

Taping Procedure:

Chronic Neck Pain General Taping Procedures:

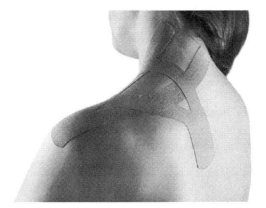 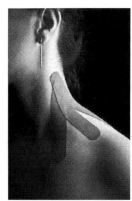

Upper Back/Mid Back Pain

Muscles to Treat (biggest troublemakers first):

1. Back Erectors
2. Trapezius
3. Rhomboids
4. Levator Scapulae
5. Serratus Posterior Superior
6. Latissimus Dorsi
7. Serratus anterior
8. Scalene group
9. Serratus Posterior Inferior
10. Infraspinatus

Kinetic Chain Stretches Needed:

1. Stretch 3
2. Stretch 4
3. Stretch 5
4. Stretch 11
5. Stretch 13
6. Stretch 17
7. Stretch 20

Common Injuries to this Area:

Thoracic Disk Bulge, T4 Syndrome, Thoracic Outlet Syndrome, Scheuermann's disease, Facet Joint Sprains

Effective Alternative Therapies:

Thoracic Disk Bulge: Chiropractic, Myofascial Release®, Active Release Technique®

T4 Syndrome: Chiropractic, Rolfing®, Active Release Technique®

Thoracic Outlet Syndrome: Chiropractic, Rolfing®, Myofascial Release®

Scheuermann's Disease: Rolfing®, Chiropractic, Any Kind of Postural Therapy Similar to Rolfing®

Facet Joint Sprains: Active Release Technique®, Graston®, Myofascial Release®

Taping Procedure:

General Taping for Upper/Mid Back Pain. Try putting tape in different areas and different angles to see what works for your case.

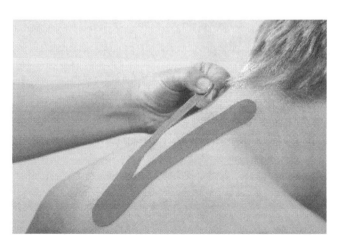

Lower Back Pain/Sciatica

Muscles to Treat (biggest troublemakers first):

1. Gluteus Medius
2. Psoas Group
3. Piriformis
4. Back Erectors
5. Quadratus Lumborum
6. Gluteus Maximus
7. Rectus Abdominis
8. Gluteus Minimus
9. Semimembranosus/Semitendinosus
10. Soleus

Kinetic Chain Stretches Needed:

1. Stretch 5
2. Stretch 6
3. Stretch 17
4. Stretch 18
5. Stretch 21
6. Stretch 20
7. Stretch 19
8. Stretch 22

Common Injuries to this Area:

Facet Joint Sprain, Lumbar Disk Bulge, Sacroiliac Joint Dysfunction, Sciatica, General Chronic Pain

Effective Alternative Therapies:

Facet Joint Sprain: Chiropractic, Graston ®, Myofacial Release Technique

Lumbar Disk Bulge: Chiropractic, Active Release Technique ®

Sacroiliac Joint Dysfunction: Chiropractic, Rolfing ®

Sciatica: Active Release Technique ®, Graston ®, Rolfing ®

General Chronic Lower Back Pain: Active Release Technique ®, Graston ®, Rolfing ®

Taping Procedure:

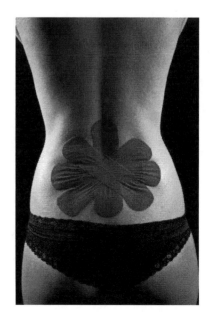

Shoulder Pain

Muscles to Treat (biggest troublemakers first):

1. Infraspinatus
2. Scalenes
3. Subscapularis
4. Teres Minor
5. Coracobrachialis
6. Supraspinatus
7. Latissimus Dorsi/ Teres Major
8. Pectoralis Major
9. Biceps Brachii
10. Trapezius
11. Serratus Anterior
12. Triceps Brachii
13. Pectoralis Minor
14. Subclavius
15. Levator Scapulae
16. Deltoid

Kinetic Chain Stretches Needed:

1. Stretch 1
2. Stretch 2
3. Stretch 7
4. Stretch 10
5. Stretch 12
6. Stretch 13
7. Stretch 14
8. Stretch 15
9. Stretch 9
10. Stretch 8

Common Injuries to this Area:

Rotator Cuff Tendonitis, Shoulder Dislocation, General Chronic Pain, Labral Tear, AC Joint Sprain, Proximal Insertion Biceptual Tendonitis

Effective Alternative Therapies:

Rotator Cuff Tendonitis: Active Release Technique ®, Graston ®, Myofascial Release ®

Shoulder Dislocation: Trigger Point Therapy, Taping

General Chronic Shoulder Pain: Active Release Technique ®, Graston ®, Myofascial Release ®, Trigger Point Therapy

Labral Tear: Graston ®, Trigger Point Therapy, Myofascial Release ®, Prolotherapy ®. Keep doing trigger point therapy at home. BE VERY CAREFUL with the kinetic chain stretches. For some people labral tears, they can help, for some, they can cause more problems. Go slow and do what feels good.

AC Joint Sprain: Active Release Technique ®, Graston ®, Myofascial Release ®

Taping Procedure:

Proximal Insertion Biceptual

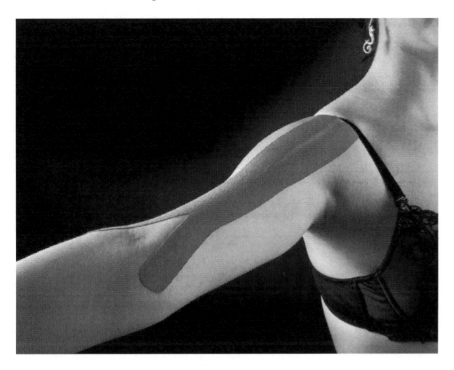

Tendonitis and general instability:

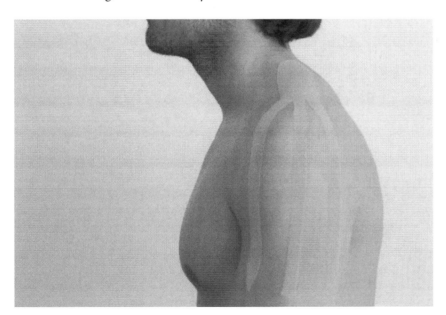

Elbow Pain

Muscles to Treat (biggest troublemakers first):
Muscles far away from the elbow that cause pain in the elbow:

1. Scalenes
2. Serratus Posterior Superior
3. Pectoralis Minor
4. Coracobrachialis
5. Infraspinatus
6. Subscapularis
7. Pectoralis Major/Minor
8. Latissimus Dorsi
9. Serratus Anterior
10. Supraspinatus

Muscles around the elbow that cause issues with the elbow:

1. Triceps Brachii
2. Biceps Brachii
3. Brachioradialis/ Extensor Carpi Radialis Group/Supinator
4. Brachialis
5. Extensor Digitorum
6. Flexor Digitorum Group/Flexor Radialis and Ulnaris

Kinetic Chain Stretches Needed:
1. Stretch 2
2. Stretch 3
3. Stretch 7
4. Stretch 10
5. Stretch 13
6. Stretch 14
7. Stretch 15
8. Stretch 16

Common Injuries to this Area:
Medial Epicondylitis, Lateral Epicondylitis, Biceps Tendonitis (Distal Insertion), Ulnar Nerve Entrapment, Triceps Tendonitis

Effective Alternative Therapies:
Medial/Lateral Epicondylitis: Graston ®, ASTYM ®, Active Release Technique ®, Rolfing ® Therapist, ESWT if severe and chronic

Biceps Tendonitis: Cross Friction Massage to tendon, ASTYM ®, Active Release Technique ®, Graston ®

Ulnar Nerve Entrapment: Active Release Technique ®, any kind of nerve mobilization therapy, Chiropractic care for unresponsive cases

Triceps Tendonitis: Graston ®, ASTYM ®, Active Release Technique ®, Rolfing ® Therapist, ESWT if severe and chronic

Taping Procedure:
Medial Epicondylitis: Put some tape on the flexor side where it hurts. Lots of methods. You can also make a "tape brace" by wrapping around the area that hurts (similar to the braces that they sell, instead you make one with athletic tape).

Triceps Tendonitis

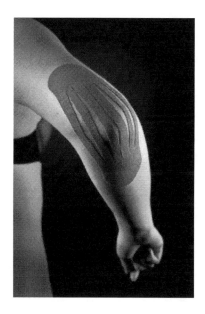

Lateral Epicondylitis

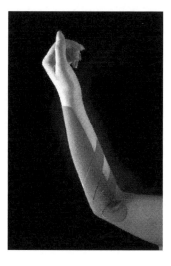
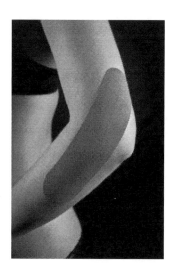

Hand/Wrist/Forearm Pain

Muscles to Treat (biggest troublemakers first):
Muscles far away from the hands/wrist and forearm that cause pain in those areas:

1. Scalenes
2. Serratus Posterior Superior
3. Pectoralis Minor
4. Triceps Brachii
5. Coracobrachialis
6. Brachialis
7. Subscapularis
8. Pectoralis Major/Minor
9. Latissimus Dorsi

Muscles near the Hands/Wrist and Forearm:

1. Brachioradialis/ Extensor Carpi Radialis Group/Supinator
2. Extensor Digitorum
3. Flexor Digitorum Group/Flexor Radialis and Ulnaris
4. Pronator Teres
5. Extensor Carpi Ulnaris
6. Flexor Hallucis Brevis
7. Opponens Pollicis/Adductor Pollicis

Kinetic Chain Stretches Needed:

1. Stretch 2
2. Stretch 3
3. Stretch 4
4. Stretch 7
5. Stretch 10
6. Stretch 13
7. Stretch 14
8. Stretch 16

Common Injuries to this Area:
Carpal Tunnel Syndrome, Finger Strain, Sprained Wrist, Sprained Thumb, Wrist Impingement,

Effective Alternative Therapies:
Carpal Tunnel Syndrome: Active Release Technique ®, Myofascial Release ®, any kind of Nerve Mobilization Therapy

Finger Strain: Graston ®, ASTYM ®, Cross Friction Massage, ESWT if severe and chronic

Sprained Wrist: When severe use a wrist splint. Graston ®, Active Release Technique ®, ESWT if severe and chronic

Sprained Thumb: Graston ®, ASTYM ®, Cross Friction Massage, ESWT if severe and chronic

Wrist Impingement: Chiropractor, Active Release Technique ®

Taping Procedure:
Finger Strain: Put a strip on the flexor side of the finger or cover the area that is damaged with tape. You can also tape one finger that is badly injured to a healthy finger next to it.

Sprained Wrist: I find that it is better to use a brace for sprained wrist. After you take off the brace (usually you should wear it for the first couple days), then you can tape the wrist. Lots of ways to do this depending on what structures you damaged. Usually you will be putting more tape on the side of the wrist that is injured. You can also wrap tape around the whole wrist and see if that helps your pain.

Perpetuating/Causative Factors:
Working at a desk

Being hunched over anything, whether it is a book, computer, desk, will cause and perpetuate Wrist/Hand and Forearm pain.

Having your hands faced downward. Lots of ergonomic inspired mice and keyboards on the market today try to put your hand and wrist in a more supinated position (facing upward).

If you depend on your hands to make money, think about what positions cause the most pain and what positions they are in throughout the day. Taking breaks consistently throughout the day to move your hands and wrists in other directions than you have them all day is a great idea. Remember that the body does not like to be in one position for very long. Try to do your work but with different hand positions/angles etc. Repetitive motions are the human body's weakness; try to avoid this problem by mixing things up often.

Hip/Buttock Pain

Muscles to Treat (biggest troublemakers first):

1. Psoas Group
2. Semimembranosus/Semitendinosus and Biceps Femoris
3. Gluteus Medius
4. Piriformis
5. Vastus Lateralis
6. Gluteus Maximus
7. Adductor Longus/Brevis and Magnus
8. Rectus Abdominis
9. Gluteus Minimus
10. Tensor Fascia Latae
11. Pectineus
12. Quadratus Lumborum

Kinetic Chain Stretches Needed:

1. Stretch 5
2. Stretch 6
3. Stretch 17
4. Stretch 18
5. Stretch 19
6. Stretch 20
7. Stretch 21
8. Stretch 22

Common Injuries to this Area:

Adductor Tendonitis, Groin Strain, Hip Flexor Strain, Quadriceps/Hamstring Strain, Buttock Pain, Glute Strain, Sciatica

Effective Alternative Therapies:

Adductor Tendonitis: ASTYM ®/Graston ®, Active Release Technique ®

Groin Strain: KT Tape®, Myofascial Release ®, Active Release Technique ®

Hip Flexor Strain: Rolfing ®, Myofascial Release ®, Active Release Technique ®

Quadriceps/Hamstring Strain: KT Tape®, Myofascial Release ®, Active Release Technique ®

Buttock Pain: Consistent Trigger Point Therapy, Rolfing ®

Glute Strain: Graston ®, Trigger point Therapy, Active Release Technique ®

Sciatica: Active Release Technique ®, Graston ®, and lots of kinetic chain stretches!

Taping Procedure:

This area is pretty tricky to tape. I suggest going to someone who knows how to tape to get it done. KT Tape® has decent techniques for taping this area. If you just throw tape on yourself, you may help the pain, but it is going to be a long shot for pain relief. I suggest not taping yourself for these injuries.

Perpetuating/Causative Factors:

- Wallet under one back pocket, this causes your hips to be shift unfavorably and predisposes you for many hip and back issues.

- Running on one side of the road makes one of the hips to be shifted higher than the other causing problems.

- Sitting all day starts a lot of issues in the hips. The hips are a very stable joint structure, but muscular problems can cause lots of pain. Keep those muscles happy by keeping them active.

- Even though you are told to have a joint replacement, most of the time you can get away with fixing the muscle dysfunctions. This is not true for everyone. Some hip issues need surgery no matter what. Be sure to ask a reputable orthopedist for their opinion.

Knee Pain

Muscles to Treat (biggest troublemakers first):

1. Vastus Lateralis/Vastus Medialis
2. Semimebranosus/Semitendinosus
3. Biceps Femoris
4. Rectus Femoris/Vastus Intermedius
5. Gastrocnemius
6. Adductor Longus/ Adductor Brevis
7. Popliteus
8. Sartorius
9. Gracilis

Kinetic Chain Stretches Needed:

1. Stretch 5
2. Stretch 6
3. Stretch 17
4. Stretch 18
5. Stretch 19
6. Stretch 20
7. Stretch 21
8. Stretch 22
9. Stretch 23

Common Injuries to this Area:

Medial/Lateral Meniscus Tear, MCL/LCL/ACL/PCL Tear, Patellofemoral Syndrome, Patellar Tendonitis, Hamstring Tendonitis, Iliotibial Band Syndrome, Quadriceps Tendonitis

Effective Alternative Therapies:

Meniscus Tears: Prolotherapy ® (very effective), PRP Injections

MCL/LCL: Graston ®/ASTYM ®, Cross Friction Massage

PCL/ACL: Orthopedist, Active Release Technique®, Lymphatic Drainage after surgery, Prolotherapy ®

Patellofemoral Syndrome: Active Release Technique®, Graston ®, ASTYM ®, Rolfing ®, Voodoo Band® to Hip and Knee muscles, Myofascial Release ®

Patellar Tendonitis: Graston ®/ASTYM ®, Cross Friction Massage, ESWT if severe and chronic

Quadriceps Tendonitis: Graston ®/ASTYM ®, Cross Friction Massage, Active Release Technique ®

Iliotibial Band Syndrome: (remember, the IT Band cannot become "tight", it exhibits symptoms due to muscular dysfunction, most of which are trigger point pain referrals). Trigger Point Therapy (professionally trained), Active Release Technique ®, Myofascial Release ®

Taping Procedure:
Iliotibial Band Syndrome:

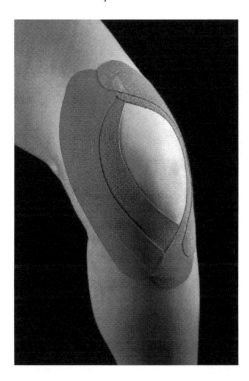

Patellofemoral Syndrome: Follow the picture above but put more tape on the lateral side. Some people try to force the patella to track more medially by pushing it over with tape. I do not think it works that way, or that is what's causing the relief. I think that the tape on the lateral side is causing a fascial release in the vastus lateralis area which is perpetuating the dysfunction. When it is released, the patella tracks more properly.

Foot Pain/Ankle Pain

Muscles to Treat (biggest troublemakers first):

1. Gastrocnemius
2. Soleus
3. Peroneal Group
4. Tibialis Anterior
5. Tibialis Posterior
6. Quadratus Plantae and other Deep Foot Flexors
7. Flexor Hallucis Brevis
8. Extensor Hallucis/Digitorum Group
9. Abductor Hallucis

Kinetic Chain Stretches Needed:

1. Stretch 6
2. Stretch 20
3. Stretch 21
4. Stretch 23
5. Stretch 24
6. Stretch 25

Common Injuries to this Area:

Plantar Fasciitis, Posterior Tibialis Tendonitis, Baxters Nerve Entrapment, Achilles Tendonitis, Ankle Instability Issues (reoccurring sprained ankles), Shin Splints, Peroneal Tendonitis, Tarsal Tunnel Syndrome

Effective Alternative Therapies:

Plantar Fasciitis/ Achilles Tendonitis: Leukotape® Taping, ESWT (extracorporeal shockwave therapy), Graston, Active Release Technique ®, ASTYM ®, Orthotic

Posterior Tibialis Tendonitis/Peroneal Tendonitis/Shin Splints: KT Tape®, Voodoo Wrap® to Calf Muscles, Orthotic, Graston®

Ankle Instability: Chiropractic Adjustments, Prolotherapy ®

Baxters Nerve Entrapment/ Tarsal Tunnel Syndrome: Active Release Technique ®, Graston ®, Myofascial Release ®, Any kind of nerve mobilization therapy

Taping Procedure:

Plantar Fasciitis:

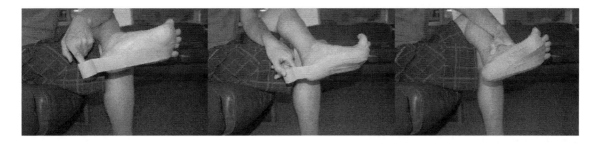

Achilles Tendonitis:

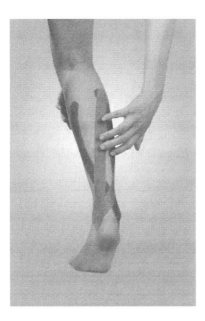

Peroneal Tendonitis:

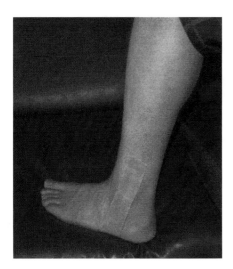

Posterior Tibialis Tendonitis:

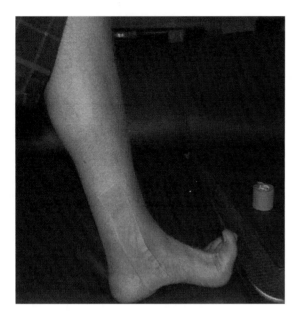

Perpetuating/Causative Factors:

Usually perpetuating and causative factors of foot pain are caused from issues in the hip. When the hip is not tilted properly, the femur does not rotate how it should, which causes the knees to come inward and makes the arches of the foot collapse. This makes the feet unable to absorb shock from the ground as efficiently and things start to break. If you have high arches and proper walking gait, you may have a bad diet or an underlying health issue. Or you are pushing it too hard in sports/exercise.

Preventative Exercises

Many injuries can be prevented if you do some exercise along with your clean diet. When the pain is gone, you will want to make sure the pain never comes back. We do this by working out any muscular imbalances. A couple muscles in the body like to become weak or inhibited and need to be worked out occasionally for proper body biomechanics.

Follow the exercises in this chapter when your pain is non-existent, or if you are a healthy individual who does not want chronic pain. Remember, these exercises do not fix a bad diet. Fix your diet, than work on these exercises.

Remember not to do these exercises until all the steps of MSTR have been applied to the muscles that you wish to strengthen for a given joint. You should only exercise when your pain is completely gone (or nearly gone, a "ghost of a pain").

None of the exercises have "sets" or "reps". Why is this so? Because everyone is different! I do not believe in training people on numbers. When I used to coach gymnastics, I would tell everyone to go as far as they could and stop. You do not need to force a muscle into extreme exhaustion to make it stronger. All you need to do is get the muscle fibers firing and give the fibers a little resistance and it will respond favorably.

If you want to train for strength or size, do more weight. If you want to train for endurance, train for longer with less weight. If you want to prevent muscle imbalances so you can get rid of chronic injury pain, you need to work out the muscle with a moderate amount of weight until the muscle is tired, and then stop.

Neck Imbalance: All-Around Neck Stability Exercise

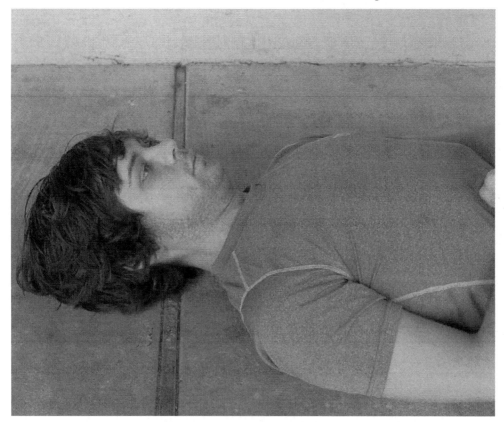

Really simple exercise. Lie on your back and lift your head a couple cm off the ground while making a double chin. This will strengthen the weak muscles in the front of your neck. Make sure you make a slight double chin. Hold the position for 30-60 seconds; less if it is difficult, more if it is easy.

Scapula Stability Imbalance: Rhomboid and Lower Trapezius Exercise

If you are an office worker who sits at a desk all day, this is an important exercise. Simply squeeze your shoulder blades together. Do it over and over until you feel a burn.

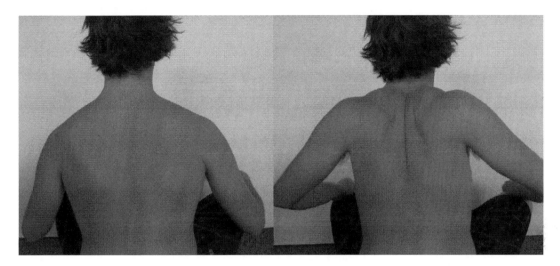

Another variation of this exercise is to lean your back flat against a wall, and squeeze your shoulder blades together.

Also you can try doing it against a wall corner. Try to squeeze the corner with your shoulder blades.

Shoulder Stability Imbalance: External Rotators of the Shoulder

Use a small weight (I am using a metal water bottle filled with sand) and assume the position in the picture below:

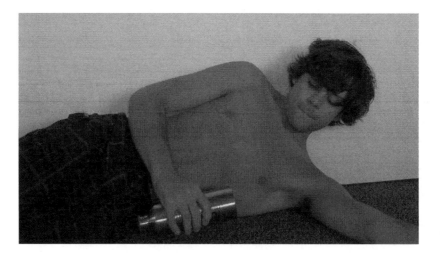

Lift up the weight while keeping your elbow against your side:

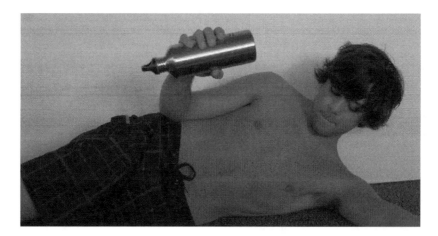

Another great option for working out these muscles is to use an exercise band. Remember to stop when the muscle is tired. You do not need to force the muscle to exhaustion to see favorable results.

Elbow Stability Imbalance: Elbow Extenders

Super simple exercise for the elbow extenders is simple cable pull downs. Assume the position in the picture below with a moderate amount of weight and pull the bar down slowly. You do not have to be big and buff or push a lot of weight. Put it on the highest amount of weight that does not cause ANY pain.

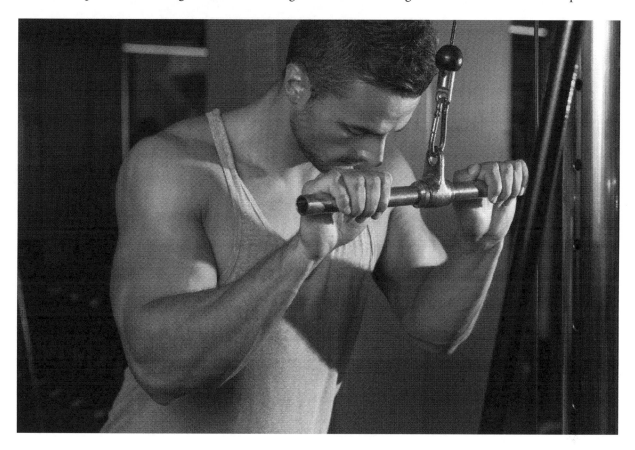

Forearm Imbalance: Weak Wrist and Hand Extensors Exercise

You can buy wrist and hand extensor workout tool available at any sports store, or you can make your very own for little to nothing!

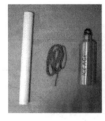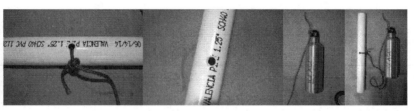

- Walk around your house and look for a cylinder shaped object. PVC pipe is super cheap and works perfectly.

- Drill a hole in the pipe, and then put a piece of string or thin rope inside the hole. Tie a knot around the hole.

- Then look around the house again for something that is 1-3 pounds. I like to use a metal water bottle filled with sand.

Now you have a new tool to work out the weak and imbalanced muscles in your forearm!

This is how you use it:

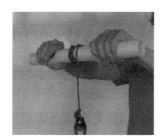

First thing to keep in mind is that you must have the weight being pulled up on the side of the pipe that is away from you (pictured above). Then you just roll the weight up and down:

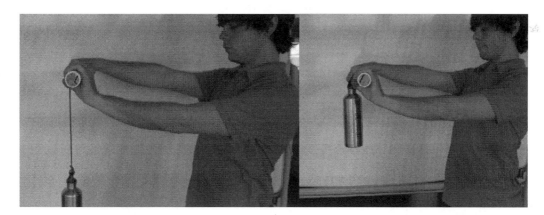

Hip Tilt Imbalance: Weak Abdominals and Glutes Exercise

Basic sit ups work well for the abdominals. There are plenty of abdominal workouts available, but sit ups are pretty decent at getting the muscles firing again and are good for anyone, regardless of health (unless you have trigger points!).

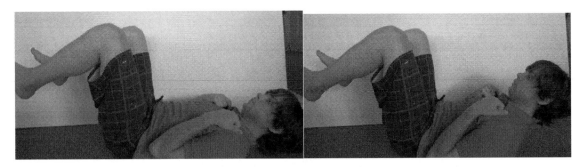

The glutes can also be trained in lots of ways, but the best way to do them if you are out of shape is by laying on your back, with your knees bent, and pushing your stomach up to the sky:

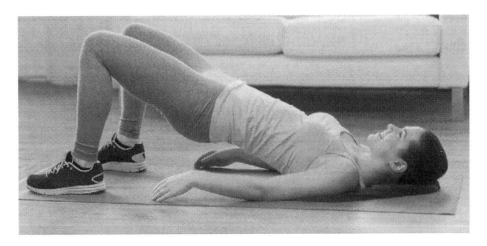

Later on you can progress to doing leg lifts with ankle weights:

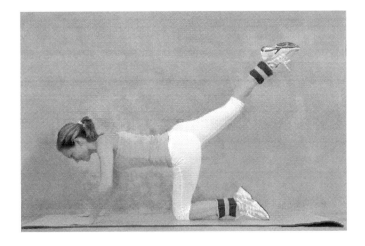

Hip Lateral Stability Imbalance: Gluteus Medius Exercise

Very simple exercise and very important for proper walking gait dynamics and so much more! Simply lie on your side, lift up your leg, and then lower it back down to the floor. If these are too hard for your, bend your knee a little bit so that you have better leverage. Most people can keep their leg straight on their first try:

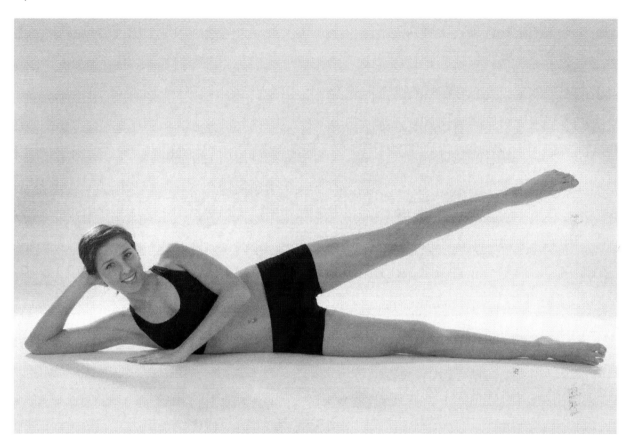

Knee Stability Imbalance: Vastus Medialis Exercise

This muscle is tricky. You must understand that the muscle is only effectively used for stabilizing the knee joint at the last 10-25 degrees of knee extension (when the knee is nearly straight). When you straighten the knee, it will be contracted fully. You can contract this muscle while standing by straightening the knees as hard as you can and feeling the location of this muscle to see how contracted it is.

One way to work this muscle out is by going on a leg lift machine (in picture below) and lifting a light weight on the last 10-25 degrees of knee extension:

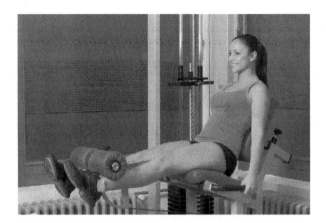

Another way is to sit on the ground, with your legs straightened as much as possible, then try to lift your heels of the ground:

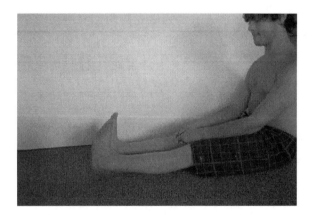

As long as you are putting resistance to the quadriceps muscle in the last 10-25 degrees of extension, you will be good to go. I also like to take a pillow case or strong bag, fill it with a little bit of sand, and use it as a weight over my ankle while I do leg lifts. A lot of weight is not important. You want to work out the muscle so that you feel a burn and then stop. We are not trying to strengthen the muscle; we want to make it fire more properly so that your posture and joint stability is more favorable.

Ankle Imbalance: Tibialis Anterior

This is a super simple exercise to fix these muscles. Stand with your back against a wall. Lean against the wall, with your knees straight and your feet about 1-2 feet away from the wall. Then lift up your feet and toes towards the sky. Lift up for a second or two, and then slowly lower down. Do these until your shins feel a good burn:

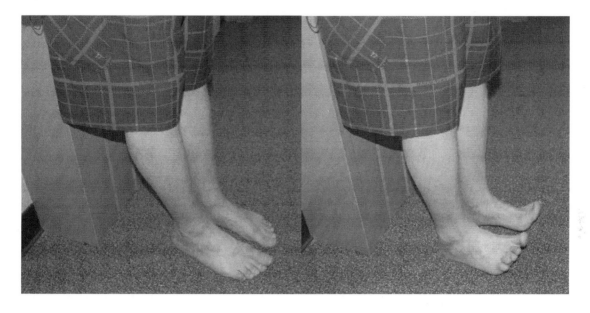

Foot Imbalance: Foot Musculature Exercise

When you are sitting down at a chair or while driving etc, lift your toes up and outward as much as possible! Make it a habit to do this when you are bored. These little muscles never get used because everyone likes to wear shoes, which makes these muscles weak and inhibited. These are crucial for long-term foot health.

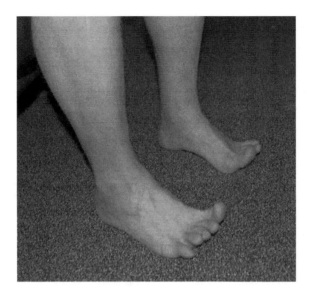

After your pain is gone, you should try to be barefoot as much as possible. This does not mean take your shoes off one day and never wear them. I mean that you should slowly progress to walking around with your shoes off more and more every day. I understand that most people cannot do this because of their jobs etc, but you need to try to make as much time as possible to being barefoot as you can. Your feet are very weak from being in shoes all your life and this can cause many problems.

In areas where people do not wear shoes, chronic foot ailments are extremely rare. We need to strengthen the foot muscles, but do so very gradually. If you take your shoes off one day and say "I am not putting them back on!" you may cause yourself some problems. So remember, progress very slowly!

Postural Considerations: Make the pain never come back!

An important thing to understand about chronic pain injuries is that they do not happen without reason. If your injury did not have a traumatic or sudden onset, less than ideal posture and dysfunctional walking gait is usually to blame. But what is "good posture"?

In order to answer this question, let's look outside of our industrialized world. I find it interesting that in countries that are not as industrialized as our own, they do not have the same posture problems we suffer with. They are also not stuck behind a desk all day, or sitting in a chair for hours on end. Body builders and fitness enthusiasts may say that you should not "squat below 90 degree knee flexion", but in some Asian countries, people pick rice all day in a so thought "unhealthy squat position" without knee problems. Some people carry baskets on their heads but do not suffer the same chronic neck pain as we do. In countries that have people walking around barefoot, there are no cases of degenerative tendonitis such as plantar fasciitis.

Why do all these people have the ability to get away with doing these "unhealthy posture" movements and have no pain? It is usually because of processed foods. If you eat processed foods when you are young and throughout your life, your body is not developed how it should be. It is extremely weak. On the other hand, indigenous people that have eaten only "unprocessed foods" have much more robust body structures. They have good posture naturally and their bones, ligaments, and muscles have adapted to whatever environment and stressors were dealt to them. They never thought "I must keep my posture good so I do not have problems later on in life", they just ate healthy foods and their body was strong enough to hold its posture on its own. Posture should not be a "conscious effort". Do you think animals go around all day thinking "I really need my posture to be good so I do not have pain"? No! This does not happen! We should eat foods that make our bodies strong, so that the body can hold its posture on its own.

You have been living your life in our industrialized world, and obviously you cannot go back in time and redevelop the dysfunctional body you are stuck in now. So you start eating healthy now, and fix your pain, but it keeps coming back. This is because the body was weak for so long (your whole life up until you started to eat healthy), that your body adapted to how weak it was (or tried to). It got by as well as it could, given its unfortunate circumstances (your processed food diet). It is still adapted to "my diet sucks and I do not have the building blocks to make this body strong, things are falling apart, but I will make them fall more slowly" mentality. The easy position that the bodies posture falls into is not a strong one.

On top of this "weakness issue" from our diet, we also have another factor to deal with in industrialized countries: Everyone sits in chairs all day. Whether we are in a car, or at work, or at home on our couch, everyone loves to sit. This makes the hips postural position unfavorable and starts the "postural problem cascade". Once the hips are out of proper alignment, everything else in the body likes to follow suit.

Because this is a long-term problem, the muscles adapt to our dysfunctional sitting habits by making some muscles shorter, and some muscles weaker. Your body figures that "I am not using a couple muscles here and a couple muscles there, so I might as well make them weaker if I am not using them! Also, some muscles are never used in their healthy range of motion, they are always shortened! I will just make them permanently shortened so that their job will be easier!" I know this all sounds scary, but these adaptations are luckily reversible!

In order to fix the misaligned posture, you must first fix the dysfunctional fascia (this substance holds your bones in their place and tells the brain what position your body is in 3 dimensional space). Rolfing ® is a great science based fascial manipulation therapy that fixes dysfunctional fascia causing bad posture. You can go to a Rolfing ® therapist, or you can stick with the kinetic chain stretches in this book and you should be good to go.

Next, you must tell the muscles what proper posture feels like. You need to train your muscles to know what proper posture is. Remember, some muscles are weak, and some are shortened. What we want to do is release the shortened muscles (with kinetic chain stretches, hopefully you have already done this earlier because of your injury, but you may need to do it some more), and then exercise the weakened muscles. This will tell the body how it should be aligned. After the body figures out "hey, this is a lot easier to support myself when my muscles are firing like this because after all, my diet is good now and it can sustain my body and make it stronger, I am going to keep my posture like this from now on!". After your body figures out what good posture is, and you continue to have a perfect diet, your posture will stay like that, without even being conscious of it.

- No processed foods for your whole life + Active lifestyle = Strong body able to support a functional posture on its own

- Over time, due to being weak from a bad diet, the body falls into the most "easiest" position which is the usual "bad posture" position (hunch back, forward shoulders, anterior pelvic tilt, knees collapsed inward etc)

- Some muscles become weak, others become shortened. This is to adapt to the new "easy" position. This puts joints into unstable position and can cause many ill effects

- In order to fix this horrible problem AFTER you have used MSTR to fix your pain: Keep eating a perfect diet, then release the dysfunctional fascia even further, where needed, then work out the muscles that are severely weakened

Where to start with good posture: The hips

The hips are your body's core. We need to start with the hips because if they are not in the proper position, everything else in the body suffers. If the hips are not in proper position, the lower spine will be curved in an unstable position. Then the legs will rotate in an unfavorable fashion, the knees will collapse inward and the arches of the foot will fall (Causing lots of problems!). The stomach will be compressed because the back is arching too much, directly causing problems with proper breathing dynamics.

How do we get the hips in an ideal position? Well first of all, let's figure out which muscles are shortened, and which ones are weakened.

Weak muscles of the hip:

- Rectus Abdominis

- Gluteus Maximus

- Gluteus Medius

Shortened muscles of the hip:

- Lower Back Erectors

- Hip Flexors: Psoas Group/Tensor Fascia Latae/Rectus Femoris

- Hamstring group

What we want to do is carefully stretch the shortened muscles with kinetic chain stretches. We also want to start working out the weak muscles. What happens when we do this is that instead of the hips being tilted forward (anterior pelvic tilt), which is seen in most people who sit down all day, the pelvis will tilt back (posterior pelvic tilt). We want to pelvis to be centered and aligned how it should, and too much anterior pelvic tilt or too much posterior pelvic tilt is bad! But what most people who sit all day have in common is that they usually have anterior pelvic tilt issues. So what we want to do is tell the body to tilt the pelvis back a little bit so that it is in proper alignment.

After you release the shortened muscles with the kinetic chain stretches as noted above, next we will work on those weak muscles. The two main muscles to think about are the Gluteus Maximus (your butt) and the Rectus Abdominis (your six pack muscles). These muscles are so weak in most people that you can barely see any definition of them at all. A lot of people in industrialized countries never have to use them and end up having no butt muscle development, and no abdominals (instead they have a big belly). What we need to do is learn how to stand and move properly so that these muscles get stronger on their own.

Your homework is to go to the "Preventative Exercises" chapter of this book and work out the muscles that are considered "weak/inhibited" for pelvic posture as noted previously.

How to stand with good pelvic posture:

Two main points. Keep your butt muscles contracted, and contract your abs a little bit. This will put the pelvis and also the spine into a proper position for stability. You can do this while walking, sitting, and standing. In order to show you how to do this, let's take a look at bad pelvic posture (anterior pelvic tilt):

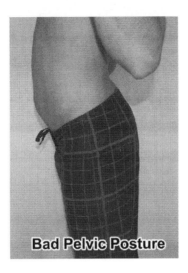

In the picture above, you can notice that the abs and glutes are not contracted, which means they are stretched and not doing their job. They are in "lazy mode". The hip flexors and back muscles on the other hand are contracted too much! This means that they are inhibited and unable to contract further, which is the perfect setup to start chronic low back pain. So let's start by contracting those abdominal muscles and gluteal muscles:

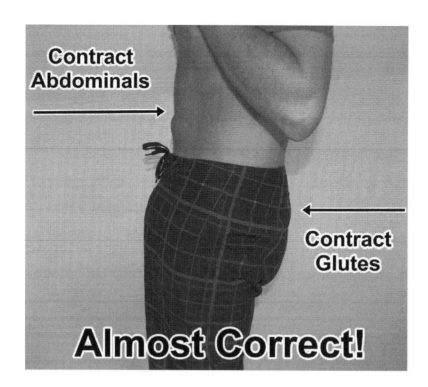

Now that we have the muscles contracted, we are almost to a good pelvic posture! All we need to do now is relax the muscles a little bit; then, you will be all good to go. The amount of contraction you should have, all day long, is 10-20 percent in your abdominals and glutes. This ensures that the muscles are doing their job. Even while writing this I have my abdominals contracted a little, and I am "pinching a penny" to keep the glutes engaged while sitting. This is what good pelvic posture looks like:

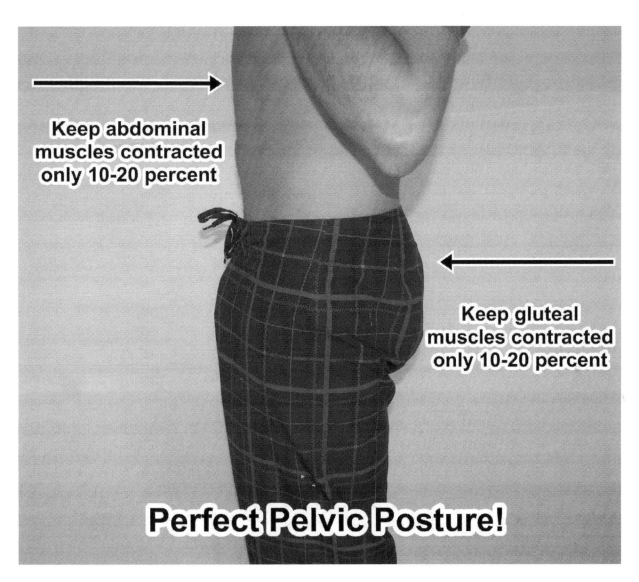

Keep abdominal muscles contracted only 10-20 percent

Keep gluteal muscles contracted only 10-20 percent

Perfect Pelvic Posture!

After a few months of having a good diet, fixing posture with MSTR, and a little contraction of the abs and glutes, you will be good to go! You won't even have to think about good pelvic posture, you will adapt to the new posture and it should stay that way.

The Next Step: Neck and Shoulder/Scapula Stability

This is very important if you work behind a desk or have a sedentary lifestyle. The neck and upper body muscles adapt in unfavorable ways for people that do not move much or are always hunched over.

You will see this in so many people when you know what to look for. It causes the head to jut forward and down (but with the chin still up), and to have the shoulders positioned more forward than they should. Over time they develop a mild "hunch back" from being bent over like this. As more time goes on, the body gets used to this position and makes it more "permanent" (a great example of this horrible posture is pictured below).

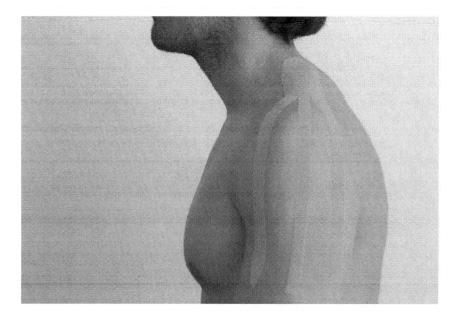

In order to fix this problem, you will fix the dysfunctional structures as noted in MSTR in the beginning of this book. After your chronic pain injures are gone, and your fascia is more adaptable due to the good diet and the kinetic chain stretches, you are now ready to fix your posture!

We will fix the neck posture by releasing some muscles even further with MSTR, and working out other muscles that are at this point weak and/or inhibited.

Weak Muscles of Dysfunctional Neck and Upper Body Posture:

- Anterior Neck Musculature

- Serratus Anterior

- Rhomboids/Lower Trapezius

- Shoulder External Rotators

Shortened Muscles of Dysfunctional Neck and Upper Body Posture:

- Posterior Neck Muscles

- Pectoralis Major/Minor

- Upper Trapezius

- Levator Scapulae

- Sternocleidomastoid

- Subscapularis/Latissimus Dorsi (Internal Rotators of Shoulder)

Your homework will be to release the muscles that are shortened by doing more MSTR to them (some of them will feel more dysfunctional than others, work on these muscles). If the muscles do not have trigger points or cross-link adhesions, skip those methods and go straight to kinetic chain stretches for each area.

After you have released those structures, which can take about two more weeks of consistent and daily effort, you are now ready to work out the weak/inhibited muscles. Head on over to the "Preventative Exercises" chapter and use the list above to strengthen the muscles that are "weak/inhibited".

After you have fixed the weak/inhibited muscles of the neck, try to keep the posture in the picture below. Imagine there being a rope attached to the top of the head, and then imagine that point being pulled upward. Also keep your shoulders back and down. After a bit of practice, you will no longer have to think about keeping this posture as it will come naturally.

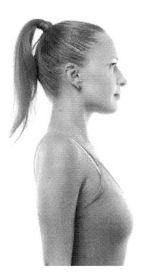

The Healing Power of Walking

You are made to walk. You are made to walk all day long, and your joints will thank you if you do. After you fix your posture/pain/diet etc, try to walk as much as possible! Walking causes nutrients to flow into your tissues, and wastes to flow out. It is very stress relieving and feels great!

Keep on walking everyday till the day you die. It helps you out mentally and physically.

Special Techniques

This section will cover what I did not cover in the previous MSTR chapters on how to mobilize soft tissue. The techniques in this section are more specialized and are usually geared at more localized mobilization methods.

Cross Friction Massage

In order to cause proliferation of fibroblasts and increased fibroblast activity, you need to perform Cross Friction Massage. Fibroblasts make scar tissue, which is needed in every injury. Even though scar tissue is "bad" in some cases, it is all we have to repair actual tears in soft tissue. In degenerative injuries, scar tissue production likes to stop. What cross friction massage aims at doing is "restarting" the inflammation process and forces the body to lay down scar tissue to fix any structural weakness in the area.

Cross Friction Massage has been around for a long time, is extremely safe, and can give you some great results. It can also be used in many areas of the body. I like using it for areas that are avascular (without blood supply) such as ligaments and sometimes in degenerative tendon issues.

If you understand how cross friction massage works, then it is easy to use anywhere in the body. All you need to know is figure out which direction the fibers are running in the degenerative structure. Most fibers are arranged in a parallel arrangement that corresponds with the lines of tensional pull that the structure has to withstand. Now what you will do is sink a small convex scrapping tool with a blunt edge into the structure. Then, instead of scraping the skin, you will rub back and forth with a good amount of effort.

What this does is cause a micro trauma that forces the body to start an inflammatory process. This inflammatory process is not degenerative, and instead is regenerative, promoting strength and healing to the area.

Tarsal Tunnel Syndrome Manual Release

The Tarsal Tunnel loves to develop pressure from chronic inflammation in the tendons that run through it. When this happens it can put pressure on the nerves and blood vessels that supply the foot. In order to release this pressure and push the metabolic wastes from this area, simply press down on the tendons and move the foot up and down. This will restore healthy movement between the structures in this area.

Median Nerve Entrapment

Most office workers get nerve entrapment to this nerve in the forearm. I am not going to go over how to mobilize a nerve in its fascial tunnel, because that is reserved for therapists that can learn the skill "hands on", in a soft tissue mobilization seminar or at a school. What you can do though is find the pronator teres and release that muscle which usually can fix the issue most of the time. The pronator teres loves to be tonus and shortened from keeping the wrist in a chronically pronated position. In order to release it, you can do the usual "trigger point" therapy, but I find that active muscular release fixes it much more easily and effectively.

In order to find the pronator teres, simply pronate your wrist and feel the area where the pronator teres is located. If you pronate the wrist, the muscle will be contracted and extremely easy to find. Then, shorten the muscle, by supinating the wrist, but keep hold of the muscle. When it is shortened you will be able to find areas of dysfunction. Press down on these areas, then slowly supinate the wrist and extend the elbow at the same time. This will cause an extreme amount of mobilization in the muscle and should fix the dysfunction pretty quickly.

If you want a step by step guide for this process, go to the muscle guide and find the pronator teres mobilization guide. Or go to http://www.mstrtherapy.com and look under treatment videos and "Hand/Wrist Pain", then find "MSTR Pronator Teres" to see a video of this being done.

Dynamic Release to Deal with Multiple Layers of Dysfunction

If you have a huge area of dysfunction or an area that has not been able to move for a long time (from being in a cast or from repetitive movement), and MSTR is not fixing the problem 100%, this method may help you. What we want is a sheering motion to break up the adhesions between the various "stuck" structures. When everything is moving again, then healing can take place much faster and function can be restored.

You need to find an area of dysfunction, press down on it with mechanical force, and then put the joints near to the area through their natural range of motion. This will cause a sheering force to break apart adhesions.

One way to do this is to modify the trigger point therapy mentioned early. If you need to use a foam roller to release a muscle or area of tissue, simply apply pressure to an area with the foam roller, then move the joints nearby and you will break up multiple layers of dysfunction. For example, while rolling out the quadriceps muscles with a foam roller, press down on an area of dysfunction and then move your knee joint while still applying pressure.

One way of causing a sheering motion is to use a Voodoo Wrap around an area of dysfunction, and then move the joints associated with the area. This is great for breaking up fascial adhesions.

Cupping to Release Superficial Fascial Adhesions

You can buy cheap Chinese cupping cups online. These tools are great for breaking up superficial fascial adhesions over a large area. Simply oil the area up (coconut oil works great), or use lotion, and put the cups on the area of dysfunction. The kind of dysfunction the Chinese cups works well to release is when the skin is tacked down. If you pinch a healthy area of your body that has not been injured, the skin will be very flexible and you can pinch it easily. In an area that has fascial adhesions, the skin will be tacked down to the underlying structures and will be extremely inflexible. What you want to do is use the cups to pull the skin off the underlying structures causing the adhesions to break. The cups use vacuum to pull the skin into the cup. You do not want to use too much vacuum. This can be easily adjusted by how many "pumps" of air you take out of the cup (usually the cups will come with a little hand pump).

After you have a few cups on an area of dysfunction, then pump the area out of the cups. Let the cups stay on the area for as long as comfortable. Some areas that are extremely dysfunctional will be hard to do and be quite painful. Keep the cups on for no more than a few minutes. If the area has been in chronic pain and it stretches over a large area, such as the lower back, then you can keep the cups on for 20 minutes. Make sure not to pump too much air out of the cups! It should be a gentle release.

Once the area is functioning after a few treatments, use the cups again, but dynamically. This way you can break up even more scar tissue adhesions. All you do is pump less air out of the cup, and move the cup over the area (while still keeping a vacuum in the cup). You will need lots of lubrication to do properly, but can be an effective means to breaking up scar tissue adhesions.

Cupping/Cross Friction Massage to Fix Superficial Scars

If you have a scar that is from a traumatic injury or surgery, you should be able to improve its functionality and appearance. There are lots of creams available to do this, but I find that many results can be found from using a combination of Chinese cupping and cross friction massage. Pretty much stick the Chinese cup right on top of the scar, then pump the air out. After that, do some transverse friction massage right on the scar. This can break up all the adhesions in and around the scar, and cause neurovascularization, which will push out metabolic waste products that have been trapped under the skin and in the scar.

TEN's Unit for Over-Activating a Muscle Causing it to Release

One interesting therapy I have found is to use a tens unit to contract a muscle that has been dysfunctional chronically. I love to do this method to big muscles, such as the glutes and the lower back musculature.

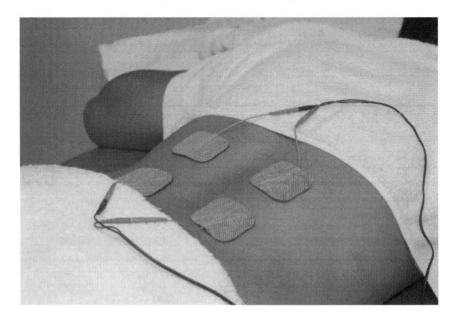

What you do is put the electrodes (sticky pads that adhere to your skin) onto a known trigger point or area of suspected dysfunctional tissue (It works better if the trigger point is huge and extremely painful). Then, turn on the tens unit and slowly put the intensity on the tens unit higher and higher until you feel a tingle. You want a decent amount of tingle, and a small amount of contraction being caused by the tens unit. Then, while wearing a glove or by covering the other side of the electrode with a cloth (something that will insulate it so as to prevent shock to your hand), massage the electrode in deep. When you move the electrode around while pushing on it, you will be able to find tender trigger points. Push the electrode into these spots and you will directly contract the trigger point (yes its already contracted, but we want to contract it more and the fibers around it so that it runs out of calcium ions and relaxes). I do not have any studies to test the validity of my claims on this method, but it works really well and is pretty safe to try on yourself.

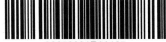

Made in the USA
San Bernardino, CA
15 January 2019